peaceful places
New York City

129 Tranquil Sites in
Manhattan, Brooklyn, Queens,
the Bronx, and Staten Island

by Evelyn Kanter

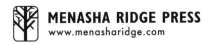

MENASHA RIDGE PRESS
www.menasharidge.com

Published by Menasha Ridge Press
Printed in the United States of America
Distributed by Publishers Group West
First edition, first printing

Cover design by Scott McGrew
Text design by Annie Long
Cartography by Steve Jones
Cover photograph by Evelyn Kanter: The Bow Bridge in Central Park,
    Upper Manhattan. See Ramble, page 128.
Unless otherwise noted, all photographs by Evelyn Kanter.
Back cover photographs by Wave Hill and Evelyn Kanter.

Library of Congress Cataloging-in-Publication Data

    Kanter, Evelyn.
        Peaceful places New York City : 129 tranquil sites in Manhattan, Brooklyn,
            Queens, the Bronx, and Staten Island / Evelyn Kanter. -- 1st ed.
            p. cm.
        ISBN-13: 978-0-89732-720-6
        ISBN-10: 0-89732-720-9
        1. New York (N.Y.)--Guidebooks. 2. Quietude. I. Title.
        F128.18.K3455 2010
        917.47'10444--dc22
                                    2009049602

Menasha Ridge Press
P.O. Box 43673
Birmingham, Alabama 35243
menasharidge.com

contents

peaceful places alphabetically

BONUS SECTION: Beyond New York City
Author's Choice: Peaceful Day Trips

dedication

To Lara and Dashiell, who give me my own peaceful places, especially when the air is singing with their giggles.

acknowledgments

*N*o project the size of this book can be researched and written without the help of friends, including the new ones you make along the way. When I told people about the theme—about quiet, tranquil, and spiritual places in a city known for its throbbing energy—everybody, without exception, offered encouragement and suggestions.

Special thanks go to John Daskalakis of the National Park Service for his knowledge about, and passion for, the wonderful nooks and crannies of the Gateway National Recreation Area and Jamaica Bay Wildlife Refuge, and to his colleague Janice Melnick for her insights about Floyd Bennett Field.

I also want to recognize the equally passionate and knowledgeable birders of the National Audubon Society. If you have the chance, grab a pair of binoculars and hike with any of them.

For ideas up and down the island of Manhattan, I send bouquets to Ed Wetschler and Susann Tepperberg—longtime friends, fellow members of the Society of American Travel Writers, and devoted residents of Greenwich Village. And to Major Gerard Fennell of the courthouse at 60 Centre Street, who does double duty as a courthouse policeman and as the historian for that landmark building.

For suggestions about their home borough of the Bronx, thanks go to two people: Bob Lape, known as the king of New York City's restaurant reviewers and my former colleague at WABC-TV and WCBS Radio news, and his wife, Joanna Pruess, the lauded chef and cookbook author.

Fellow journalist Kate McLeod, a recent transplant from Manhattan to Brooklyn, helped me focus on the very best peaceful places in her new home borough.

My son, Gerry Kanter, shared with me many favorite spots in his adopted home borough of Queens. Ditto for Queens' Robert Sinclair, who enjoys his borough's parks when he isn't test-driving cars for AAA.

On Staten Island, Pat Wilks of the Staten Island Borough President's office offered good suggestions to add to my knowledge of her part of New York City.

In addition, General Motors and Ford Motor Company graciously loaned me current model vehicles with accurate dashboard navigation systems that allowed me to find still more hidden spots in comfort and luxury. That helped immensely for my research to locate the best places for you. However, with each entry, I include information about public transportation, which is how I typically travel around New York myself.

Another debt of appreciation goes to all the Urban Park Rangers, as well as those New York City Department of Parks & Recreation workers, local residents, and office workers I met along the way who generously shared information and directions, but not their names. You know who you are!

And last but not least, thanks go to Menasha Ridge Press publisher Bob Sehlinger, who developed the concept for this book. May it guide you to many, many peaceful places that you will treasure over and over again.

Evelyn Kanter
New York
February 2010

three paths to 129 peaceful places

eaceful Places: New York City takes you to 129 tranquil sites in Manhattan, Brooklyn, Queens, the Bronx, and Staten Island. In fact, author Evelyn Kanter serves up 129 locales throughout the five boroughs, plus another four in Beyond New York City (see page 178). To make it easy for you to find an entry that suits your mood and desired neighborhood or type of place, we have organized the sites in three different ways:

first path ALPHANUMERICALLY

Each entry unfolds in the main text, beginning on page 3, in alphabetical order and is numbered in sequence. The number travels with that entry throughout the book—in the Table of Contents (page v), in the Peaceful Places by Area guide (page xv), in the Peaceful Places by Category guide (page xix), and on the main maps (pages xxv–xxxiii). (The bonus map and text, pages 178–182, are not numbered.)

second path BY AREA

The Peaceful Places by Area guide—and maps—locate sites according to these eight geographic breakouts: Northern Manhattan, Upper Manhattan, Midtown Manhattan, Lower Manhattan, Brooklyn, Queens, the Bronx, and Staten Island.

third path BY CATEGORY

The Peaceful Places by Category guide showcases the sites as listed below. In many cases it was difficult to categorize a place, as it might be a historic site in an outdoor habitat with a scenic vista that feels like a spiritual enclave that is an urban surprise where you can take an enchanting walk! But we tagged each of the 129 sites as seemed most fitting for the focus of the author's description:

Enchanting Walks	Outdoor Habitats	Reading Rooms	Spiritual Enclaves
Historic Sites	Parks & Gardens	Scenic Vistas	Urban Surprises
Museums & Galleries	Quiet Tables	Shops & Services	

PEACEFULNESS RATINGS

At the top of the main text for each profile, boxed information notes the entry's type of place, as described above. This capsule information also includes the author's rating for the site on a scale of one to three stars, as follows:

✪ ✪ ✪   Heavenly anytime

✪ ✪   Almost always sublime

✪   Tranquil if visited as described in the entry—during times of day, week, season, etc.—and possibly avoided at certain times

—The Publisher

peaceful places by area

NORTHERN MANHATTAN
(110th Street to the northern tip of the island)

UPPER MANHATTAN
(59th Street to 110th Street)

MIDTOWN MANHATTAN
(23rd Street to 59th Street)

LOWER MANHATTAN
(23rd Street to the Battery)

BROOKLYN

BRONX

STATEN ISLAND

BONUS SECTION: Beyond New York City
Author's Choice: Peaceful Day Trips

peaceful places by category

ENCHANTING WALKS

PARKS & GARDENS

PARKS & GARDENS (*continued*)

QUIET TABLES

READING ROOMS

SCENIC VISTAS

SHOPS & SERVICES

SPIRITUAL ENCLAVES

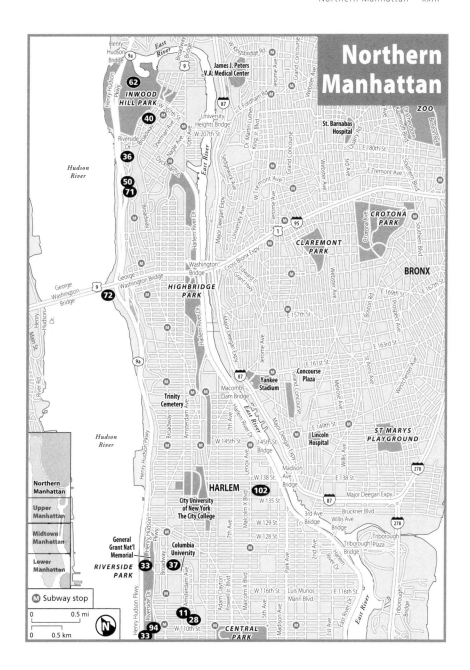

Northern Manhattan

Henry Hudson Bridge — 9a
East River
W. Kingsbridge Rd.
Broadway
9
James J. Peters V.A. Medical Center
Grand Concourse
Webster Ave.
ZOO
Dr. Theodore Kazmiroff Blvd.
Boston Rd.
62
INWOOD HILL PARK
Henry Hudson Pkwy.
87
University Heights Bridge
E. Fordham Rd.
Jerome Ave.
St. Barnabas Hospital
Southern Blvd.
40
W. 207th St.
Dr. Martin Luther King Jr. Blvd.
3rd Ave.
E. 180th St.
E. Tremont Ave.
Riverside Dr.
Sherman Ave.
10th Ave.
36
Dyckman St.
Naegle Ave.
Broadway
W. Tremont Ave.
Major Deegan Expy.
Jerome Ave.
Webster Ave.
Hudson River
50
71
Harlem River Dr.
East River
University Ave.
Jerome Ave.
CROTONA PARK
Crotona Ave.
Southern Blvd.
Broadway
1
95
CLAREMONT PARK
Webster Ave.
BRONX
E. 169th St.
E. 167th St.
George Washington Bridge
9
Washington Bridge
George Washington Bridge
HIGHBRIDGE PARK
Cross Bronx Expy.
Edward L. Grant Hwy.
Boston Rd.
Prospect Ave.
St. Ann's Ave.
Westchester Ave.
72
Harlem River Dr.
E. 157th St.
E. 163rd St.
Henry Hudson Dr.
River Rd.
Henry Hudson Pkwy.
9a
Major Deegan Expy.
Jerome Ave.
E. 161st St.
Grand Concourse
Concourse Plaza
Melrose Ave.
87
Yankee Stadium
Macombs Dam Bridge
Trinity Cemetery
Amsterdam Ave.
Broadway
Harlem River Dr.
East River
E. 149th St.
Lincoln Hospital
Willis Ave.
ST. MARYS PLAYGROUND
Hudson River
W. 145th St.
145th St. Bridge
2nd Ave.
278
Henry Hudson Pkwy.
Lenox Ave.
Madison Ave. Bridge
E. 138 St.
Major Deegan Expy.
278
W. 138 St.
102
Northern Manhattan
HARLEM
Malcolm X Blvd.
W. 135 St.
3rd Ave. Bridge
Bruckner Blvd.
Willis Ave. Bridge
Upper Manhattan
City University of New York The City College
7th Ave.
W. 129 St.
W. 128 St.
Park Ave.
Triborough Plaza
Triborough Bridge
Midtown Manhattan
General Grant Nat'l Memorial
Columbia University
Adam Clayton Powell Jr. Blvd.
Malcolm X Blvd.
5th Ave.
Madison Ave.
Lower Manhattan
33
37
W. 116th St.
Luis Munos Marin Blvd.
E. 116th St.
1st Ave.
Harlem River Dr.
East River
Triborough Bridge
Henry Hudson Pkwy.
Riverside Dr.
RIVERSIDE PARK
Broadway
Amsterdam Ave.
M Subway stop
11
28
94
W. 110th St.
CENTRAL PARK
33
0   0.5 mi
0   0.5 km
N

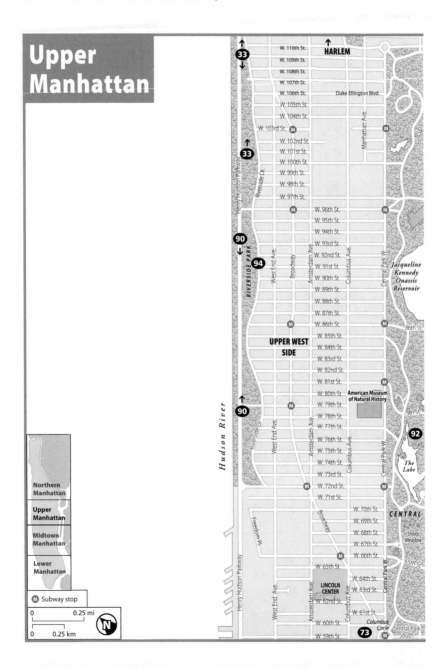

Upper Manhattan

W. 110th St.
W. 109th St.
W. 108th St.
W. 107th St.
W. 106th St.   Duke Ellington Blvd.
W. 105th St.
W. 104th St.
W. 103rd St.
W. 102nd St.
W. 101st St.
W. 100th St.
W. 99th St.
W. 98th St.
W. 97th St.
W. 96th St.
W. 95th St.
W. 94th St.
W. 93rd St.
W. 92nd St.
W. 91st St.
W. 90th St.
W. 89th St.
W. 88th St.
W. 87th St.
W. 86th St.
W. 85th St.
W. 84th St.
W. 83rd St.
W. 82nd St.
W. 81st St.
W. 80th St.
W. 79th St.
W. 78th St.
W. 77th St.
W. 76th St.
W. 75th St.
W. 74th St.
W. 73rd St.
W. 72nd St.
W. 71st St.
W. 70th St.
W. 69th St.
W. 68th St.
W. 67th St.
W. 66th St.
W. 65th St.
W. 64th St.
W. 63rd St.
W. 62nd St.
W. 61st St.
W. 60th St.
W. 59th St.

HARLEM

UPPER WEST SIDE

CENTRAL

Jacqueline Kennedy Onassis Reservoir

American Museum of Natural History

The Lake

Sheep Meadow

LINCOLN CENTER

Columbus Circle

Central Park South

Hudson River

Henry Hudson Parkway

Riverside Dr.

RIVERSIDE PARK

West End Ave.

Broadway

Amsterdam Ave.

Columbus Ave.

Manhattan Ave.

Central Park W.

Freedom Pl.

86th St.

79th St.

65th St.

33
33
90
94
90
92
73

Northern Manhattan
Upper Manhattan
Midtown Manhattan
Lower Manhattan

Subway stop

0   0.25 mi
0   0.25 km

N

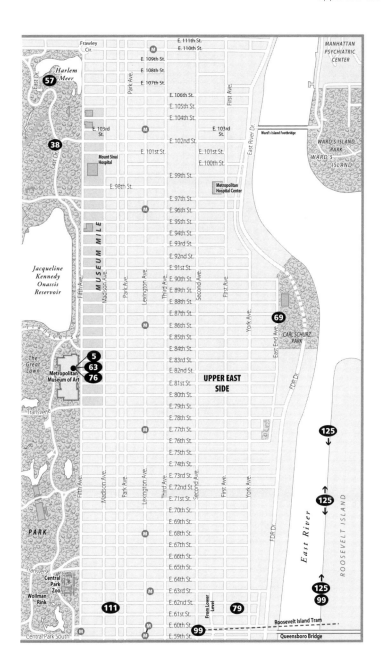

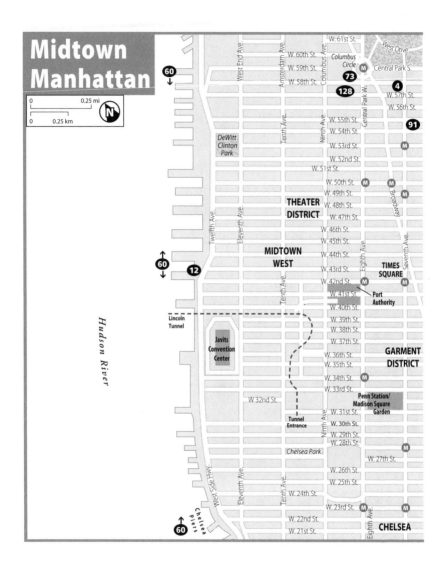

Midtown Manhattan

0   0.25 mi
0   0.25 km

N

Hudson River

West End Ave.
Amsterdam Ave.
Columbus Ave.
Central Park W.
Tenth Ave.
Ninth Ave.
Twelfth Ave.
Eleventh Ave.
Tenth Ave.
Eighth Ave.
Seventh Ave.
Broadway
Ninth Ave.
Eleventh Ave.
Tenth Ave.
Eighth Ave.
West Side Hwy.

W. 61st St.
West Drive
W. 60th St.
W. 59th St.   Columbus Circle   Central Park S.
W. 58th St.
W. 57th St.
W. 56th St.
W. 55th St.
W. 54th St.
W. 53rd St.
W. 52nd St.
W. 51st St.
W. 50th St.
W. 49th St.
W. 48th St.
W. 47th St.
W. 46th St.
W. 45th St.
W. 44th St.
W. 43rd St.
W. 42nd St.
W. 41st St.   Port Authority
W. 40th St.
W. 39th St.
W. 38th St.
W. 37th St.
W. 36th St.
W. 35th St.
W. 34th St.
W. 33rd St.
W. 32nd St.
W. 31st St.
W. 30th St.
W. 29th St.
W. 28th St.
W. 27th St.
W. 26th St.
W. 25th St.
W. 24th St.
W. 23rd St.
W. 22nd St.
W. 21st St.

DeWitt Clinton Park

THEATER DISTRICT

MIDTOWN WEST

TIMES SQUARE

Lincoln Tunnel

Javits Convention Center

GARMENT DISTRICT

Penn Station/ Madison Square Garden

Tunnel Entrance

Chelsea Park

CHELSEA

Chelsea Piers

60   73   128   4   91   12   60   60

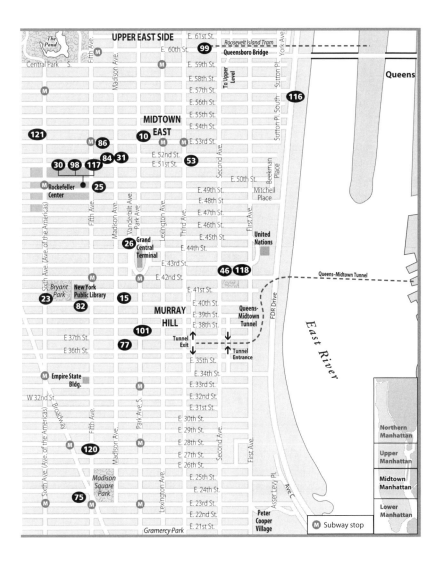

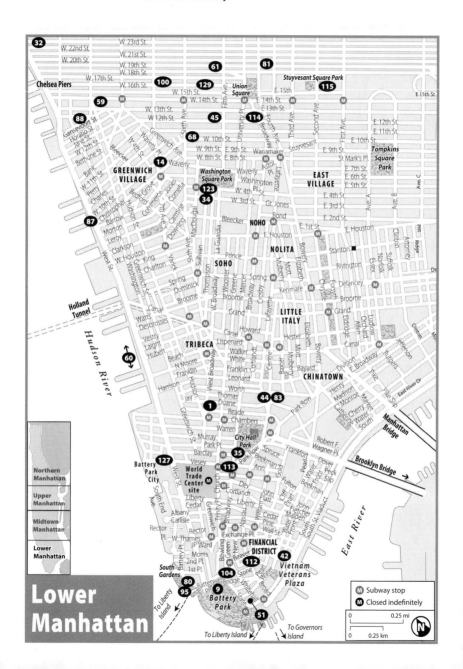

Lower Manhattan

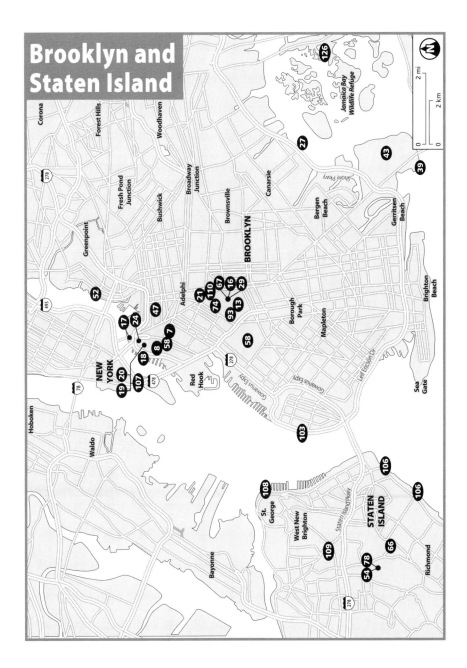

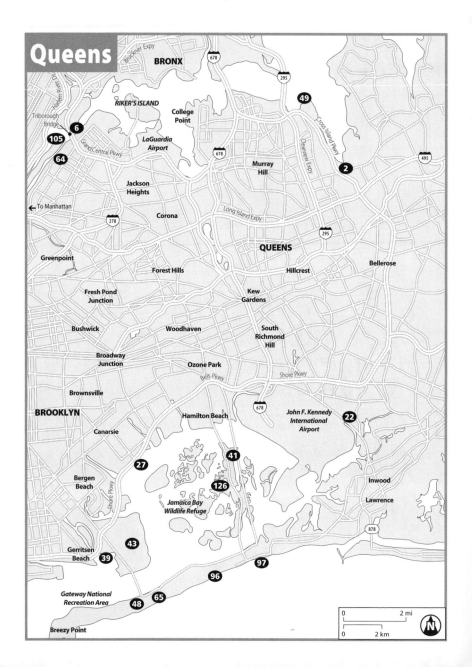

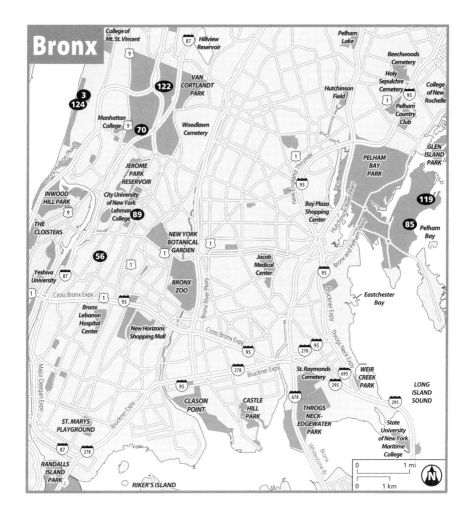

have lived in New York City all my life, and I am convinced that it is the most vibrant, fascinating, creative, diverse, and, sometimes, frustrating place on earth. Before researching and writing *Peaceful Places*, I also thought I knew my city well. After all, I had scoured its corners first with my parents, then with my children, and then for many years as a beat reporter for the evening news.

However, collecting ideas for this book gave me the opportunity to visit some spots I just never got to before—the ones on the "next week" list that never seemed to make it to the "today" list. Plus, I had the joy of returning to places I hadn't visited in what seems like a lifetime. One that I am sharing with you is what I used to call my secret garden, in Northern Manhattan's Inwood neighborhood. My junior high school was across the street from what was then known simply as the Dyckman House (now Dyckman Farmhouse Museum, described on page 57), and I often did my homework in the garden behind the historic, landmark building.

In creating this book, I was reminded that we all need tranquility and serenity in our lives. I love to surprise visitors, new transplants, and even longtime residents by describing the wealth of quiet, often spiritual, places and spaces within New York's five boroughs and along its magnificent waterways. Here, in a city known for five-star prices that match its five-star energy, you'll find many free hideaways and activities, from smelling the flowering profusion in the Brooklyn Botanic Garden to pedaling your bike on a boardwalk that borders the Atlantic Ocean.

You will also be pleased to see that nearly all of these sites are easily accessible by public transportation. That is always the best way to get around this traffic-jammed metropolis. Where else but in New York City can you take the subway to the ocean?

As described in the earlier section Three Paths to 129 Peaceful Places, the entries are listed alphabetically, as well as cross-referenced in the front by category and by location. This arrangement makes it easy for residents and visitors alike to use the book. If you're in the mood for a garden setting one day but a quiet cafe table the next, you will find the perfect place in this book.

In closing, I'll say that I chose my 129 sites (plus the 4 locations in the bonus section, Beyond New York City) anticipating that you locals will discover wonderful new spots for renewing your spirit. May this book encourage you to reaffirm your love affair with the Big Apple.

And for visitors, I especially set out to show that New York City is much more than concrete, skyscrapers, and noise. After you have explored all of the exciting tourist highlights, there are acres and acres of natural, quiet, scenic, and protected places that will welcome you with their beauty and peacefulness.

After all, from Manhattan, to Brooklyn, to Queens, to the Bronx, to Staten Island— New York City can be a peaceful, tranquil place. You just have to know where to look.

Evelyn Kanter
New York
February 2010

peaceful place 1

AFRICAN BURIAL GROUND NATIONAL MONUMENT
Lower Manhattan

CATEGORY ✌ spiritual enclaves ✪

*I*n 1991, when construction workers were excavating this corner for a new office building across the street from the U.S. Courthouse at Foley Square, they stumbled upon the remains of 419 souls, including young children. This land had been part of what was known originally as the Negroes Burying Ground, where slaves and freed slaves were laid to rest, starting in the late 1600s. The discovered remains were transferred to Howard University, in Washington, D.C., for study before being reinterred at this corner of Broadway and Duane streets, which was turned over to the National Park Service. Except for Black History Month in February and Kwanzaa in December, it is always quiet here. Office workers, attorneys, and jurors tend to rush past, ignoring the perfect green lawn and gently gurgling waterfall. The small burial-ground park features a striking black marble semicircle. It is carved with African symbols, which you can view as you walk the gently sloping path between the street level and the burial level. Among the symbols is the heart-shaped Akoma, representing patience and tolerance. There's also a steeply slanted black marble A-frame that you can enter. Like the semicircle, it has one side at street level and the other side connected to steps to the burial level. It is dark and hushed inside, inspiring meditation or, perhaps, a prayer of remembrance.

✌ essentials

290 Broadway Street (at Duane Street), Manhattan 10007

(212) 637-2019

nps.gov/afbg or africanburialground.gov

$ Free admission

🕐   Open daily, 9 a.m.–5 p.m. (except on federal holidays); 9 a.m.–4 p.m. during winter.

🚌   **By subway:** J, M, or Z to Chambers Street; 4, 5, or 6 to City Hall.

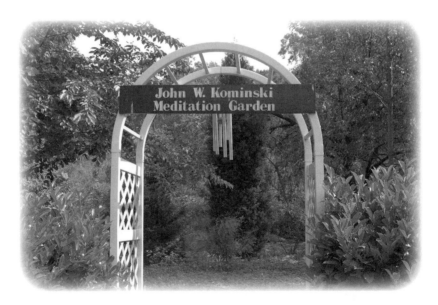

One of the author's favorite spots at Alley Pond Environmental Center

peaceful place 2

ALLEY POND ENVIRONMENTAL CENTER
Douglaston, Queens

CATEGORY ༀ outdoor habitats ✪ ✪

Giant elms, birches, and willows frame the two walking trails here, one wooded, the other marshier. The Cat Trail is a half-mile loop along a wood-chip and grass path. Part of the trail parallels the busy Cross Island Parkway a few dozen yards away, but if you are here when there are leaves on the trees, the thick foliage muffles both the sound and the sight of traffic. The trail also passes a small pond, where benches in a clearing beckon you to sit and listen to the bullfrogs and watch the mallards. The Windmill Trail is named for the city's only working windmill, built to draw water for the former farmland here. This trail also has a small meditation garden that invites you to pause and enjoy reflection. Because this educational center is popular with school groups on weekday mornings and with families on weekends, the best time to visit is weekday afternoons.

ༀ essentials

✉ 228-06 Northern Boulevard, Douglaston, Queens 11363

☎ (718) 229-4000   🌐 alleypond.com $ Free admission

🕐 Nature Center: Monday–Saturday, 9 a.m.–4:30 p.m.; Sunday, 9 a.m.–3:30 p.m.
Closed Sundays in July and August. Trails: open daily, sunrise to sunset.

🚇 **By subway:** 7 to Main Street, then the Q12 bus to Northern Boulevard (East).
Or take the Long Island Rail Road to Bayside, and walk south to Northern Boulevard
for the Q12 bus.

AQUATIC GARDEN AND PERGOLA, WAVE HILL
Bronx
CATEGORY ⌒ parks & gardens ✪ ✪

*W*ave Hill, a 28-acre public garden, has graceful wooden benches that line the garden's large lily pond, so you can sit and listen to the bullfrogs and watch the hummingbirds and butterflies. In summer, the pond also sprouts feathery reeds and other aquatic plants. Their dancelike waving to even the slightest breeze always fascinates me. More benches line the weathered wooden pergola that borders this garden. It is favored by strolling couples, their hands intertwined much like the wisteria vines that decorate it.

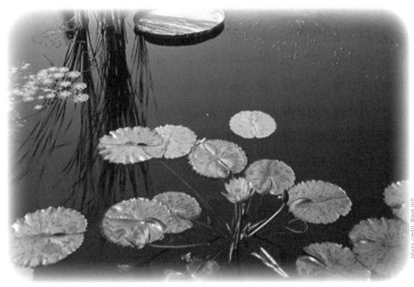

photo credit: Wave Hill

The aquatic garden at Wave Hill in the Bronx

⌣ essentials

675 West 252nd Street (entrance at West 249th Street and Independence Avenue), Bronx 10471

(718) 549-3200

wavehill.org

$ Adult admission $6; seniors and students $3; children age 6 and up $2; free until noon on Tuesdays and Saturdays year-round and all day Tuesdays during January–April, July–August, and November–December

April 15–October 14: Tuesday–Sunday, and some holiday Mondays, 9 a.m.–5:30 p.m.; October 15–April 14: Tuesday–Sunday, and some holiday Mondays, 9 a.m.–4:30 p.m.; June–July, to 8:30 p.m. on Wednesdays.

By subway: 1 to West 242nd Street, then take the free shuttle service to and from Wave Hill; call or check the Web site for the shuttle schedule.
By bus: Take the BxM1 Express bus from Manhattan's East Side, or the BxM2 bus from Manhattan's West Side. **By train:** Take the Metro-North train to Riverdale, then take the free shuttle service to and from Wave Hill; call or check the Web site for the shuttle schedule.

peaceful place 4

ART STUDENTS LEAGUE
Midtown Manhattan

CATEGORY ⌣ museums & galleries ✪

*S*ince 1892, this town house has drawn art teachers and students from around the world: Alexander Calder, Georgia O'Keeffe, Thomas Hart Benton, Red Grooms, and Augustus Saint-Gaudens have been among the league's participants. Exhibits in the large second-floor gallery change weekly from January to May, featuring the works of one student class, then another. Watercolors dominate one week, kinetic art or bronze sculptures another, so part of the enjoyment is the delight at finding something personally meaningful from an emerging artist. And, of course, the works are available for purchase. You might be bringing home the next Picasso.

⌣ essentials

✉	215 West 57th Street (at Seventh Avenue), Manhattan 10019
✆	(212) 247-4510
🌐	theartstudentsleague.org
$	Free admission
🕐	Monday–Friday, 9 a.m.–8:30 p.m.; Saturday, 9 a.m.–3 p.m.
🚃	**By subway:** 1, A, B, C, or D to 59th Street/Columbus Circle; N, Q, R, or W to 57th Street/Seventh Avenue.

peaceful place 5

ASTOR COURT, METROPOLITAN MUSEUM OF ART
Upper East Side, Upper Manhattan
CATEGORY ↙ museums & galleries ✪ ✪ ✪

*N*amed for philanthropist and benefactor Brooke Astor and her husband's Vincent Astor Foundation, this courtyard is a re-creation of a Ming Dynasty (1368–1644) garden from the city of Souzhou, near Shanghai, known for its garden architecture. An inscription above one entrance translates to—appropriately—"in search of quietude," and you'll discover it here, surrounded by ornately carved furniture, ceramics, and lacquers from China, Korea, and Japan. Some might find the small court-yard claustrophobic, but its intimate scale is a major part of its charm, and also why it's rarely crowded. My mother was a milliner who took pride in her precise stitching, so I find special solace in the heavily embroidered silks and other textiles on display in the Asian galleries around the Astor Court.

↙ essentials

≡   1000 Fifth Avenue (at 82nd Street), Manhattan 10028

℮   (212) 535-7710   ⊕   metmuseum.org

$ Adult admission $20; seniors $15; students $10; free for members and children under 12 accompanied by an adult

🕐   Tuesday–Thursday, 9:30 a.m.–5:30 p.m.; Friday–Saturday, 9:30 a.m.–9 p.m.; Sunday, 9:30 a.m.–5:30 p.m.; open some holiday Mondays.

🚌   **By subway** from the East Side of Manhattan: 4, 5, or 6 to 86th Street, and walk three blocks west to Fifth Avenue. **By bus:** M1, 2, 3, or 4 to 82nd Street. **By subway** from the West Side of Manhattan: 1 to 86th Street, then the M86 bus across Central Park to Fifth Avenue; C train to 81st Street, then the M79 bus across Central Park to Fifth Avenue.

peaceful place 6

ASTORIA PARK
Astoria, Queens
CATEGORY ↝ parks & gardens ✪ ✪

*L*ocal residents, including my son, call the mile-long Shore Road "the strip," since it is as close as 21st-century New York City gets to the parade of hot rods and crowds of onlookers that defined Hollywood's version of the 1950s. But only on weekend evenings. The rest of the time, this 65-acre oasis of breezy green along the East River, between the Queens anchors of the Robert F. Kennedy/Triborough Bridge and

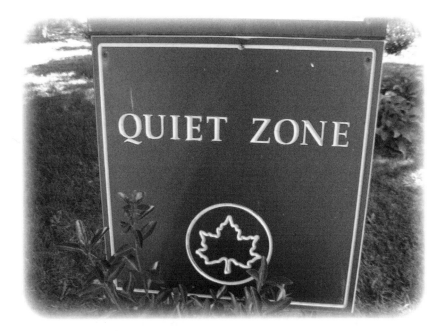

In Astoria Park next to the memorial to World War I soldiers

Amtrak's Hell Gate Bridge, offers your choice of a broad, open lawn and little enclaves of tall trees providing shade, all with spectacular views of Manhattan. This part of the river, known as Hell Gate, is fraught with treacherous currents; it was the site of the 1904 disaster that killed 1,021 people when the steamboat *General Slocum* caught fire. That was considered to be the city's worst single disaster until the World Trade Center nightmare of September 11, 2001, but this place still offers a sense of serenity. My preferred spot for contemplation is the meditation circle of large rocks (small boulders?) in the marked Quiet Zone next to the memorial to Long Island's World War I soldiers, at the southern end of the park.

essentials

East River to 19th Street, between Hoyt Avenue and Ditmars Boulevard; Queens 11102

(212) 639-9675

nycgovparks.org/parks/astoriapark

Free admission

Open daily, 6 a.m.–1 a.m.

By subway: N or W to Astoria Boulevard or Ditmars Boulevard, and walk west five minutes to the park. **By bus:** Q19A to Hoyt Avenue.

peaceful place 7

ATLANTIC AVENUE
Brooklyn Heights, Brooklyn

CATEGORY ↷ enchanting walks ✪

*D*espite the fact that this bustling thoroughfare anchors the commercial heart of Brooklyn Heights and its northern border, you can turn it into your own private mecca. Just set your mind to leisurely browsing and sampling at Sahadi's Specialty and Fine Foods—187 Atlantic Avenue, (718) 624-4550, sahadis.com, Monday–Saturday, 9 a.m.–7 p.m. Dreamily, you can transport yourself to the Old World Middle East. Wooden shelves groan under cans and jars bearing Arabic labels. Barrels with dozens of varieties of green and ripe olives sit alongside yawning sacks of dried apricots, coffee beans, and long- and short-grain rices. The aromas tempt the senses and the shopping bag. It is impossible not to nibble, and once you do, you will be swooping up a half-pound of this and a full pound of that. Who knew there were so many varieties of lentils? But the point is to do so in a state of tranquility, not with a must-do shopping list in your hands.

The yin to Sahadi's yang is Damascus Bread and Pastry, a few doors away— 195 Atlantic Avenue, (718) 625-7070, open daily, 7 a.m.–7:30 p.m. Damascus tempts you with homemade meat pies, fresh balls of falafel waiting to be stuffed into a fresh-baked pita, and trays of baklava and other delicate pastries with crushed pistachios, honey, and chopped dates. Gather items from Sahadi's and Damascus for a picnic lunch to enjoy on your stroll along the Brooklyn Heights Esplanade (see page 26).

✨ essentials

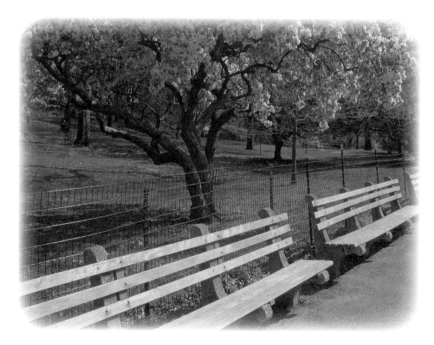 Atlantic Avenue, Henry Street to Court Street; Brooklyn 11201

✆ No phone

🌐 nycvisit.com

$ Free admission

🕐 Open daily, hours vary

🚃 **By subway:** 2, 3, M, or R to Court Street; A, C, or F to Jay Street/Borough Hall.

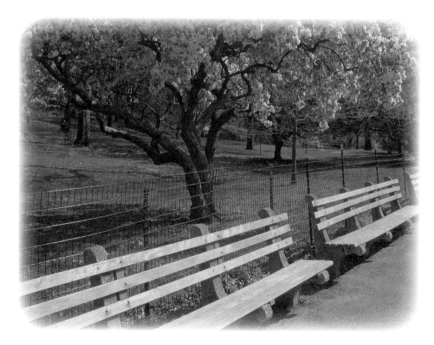

Old-fashioned stone-and-wood benches abound in New York City parks.

peaceful place 8

ATLANTIC BOOKSHOP
Brooklyn Heights, Brooklyn
CATEGORY ⤙ shops & services ✪ ✪

*Y*ou never know what you'll find in this eclectic secondhand bookshop. Although it specializes in out-of-print academia, bookshelves also groan with a wealth of rare leather-bound first editions and current novels. The day I visited, I respectfully held a two-volume *Commentary on the Apocalypse* by Moses Stewart printed in 1845.

⤙ essentials

✉	179 Atlantic Avenue, Brooklyn 11201
✆	(718) 797-5756
🌐	abebooks.com/servlet/StoreFrontDisplay?cid=91097
$	Free admission
🕐	Monday–Thursday, 10 a.m.–8 p.m.; Friday–Saturday, 11 a.m.–7 p.m.; Sunday, 10 a.m.–7 p.m.
🚇	**By subway:** 2, 3, 4, 5, or R to Court Street/Borough Hall; A, C, or F to Jay Street/Borough Hall; F to Bergen Street.

peaceful place 9

BATTERY PARK AND CASTLE CLINTON NATIONAL MONUMENT

Lower Manhattan

CATEGORY ⌣ parks & gardens ✪ ✪

ou could call this Manhattan island's big green toe, a giant lawn dotted with mature trees, sculptures, and monuments. An imposing arrangement of marble towers is carved with the names of New York City's World War II servicemen and women. From here you will enjoy spectacular views across New York Harbor to the Statue of Liberty and Ellis Island. A wall of benches lines the water, but tourists waiting for the ferries to Miss Liberty and Ellis Island almost always dilute the panorama. My choice for a secluded bench is to walk inland on the lawn, but in good weather I make sure that I go there before or after the peak lunch hours, when the park is picnic central for nearby office workers. In overcast or cool weather, it is possible to snag a good vantage point in your own private square of lawn. Ready to move again? Then take a few minutes to wander through Castle Clinton, a small circular fort built to defend the harbor just before the War of 1812, now part of the National Park System.

⌣ essentials

⊞ State Street and Battery Place, Manhattan 10004

☏ Battery Park: (212) 344-3491; Castle Clinton: (212) 344-7220

🌐 thebattery.org; nps.gov/cacl

$ Free admission

🕐 Park: open daily, 6 a.m.–1 a.m. Castle Clinton: open daily, 8:30 a.m.–5 p.m.

🚌 **By subway:** 1 to South Ferry; 4 or 5 to Bowling Green; R or W to Whitehall Street. **By ferry:** Staten Island Ferry to Battery Park. **By bus:** M1, 6, or 15 to Battery Park.

peaceful place 10

BAUMAN RARE BOOKS
Midtown Manhattan

CATEGORY ⤳ shops & services ✪ ✪ ✪

*P*art bookstore, part gallery, this is the place to come for hushed tomes, burnished wood shelves, and elegant Oriental carpeting. The sight of row upon row of gold-embossed leather-bound books slows me down instantly. Ditto as I wander by showcases of historic autographs and other memorabilia depicting the lives of authors and composers. Where else would you expect to find Beethoven, ancient Bibles and Torahs, Mark Twain, and a signed first edition of an Ian Fleming James Bond novel, all in one place? Better yet, the staff recognizes the difference between a browser and a buyer—and both are made to feel very welcome.

⤳ essentials

🖃 535 Madison Avenue (at 54th Street), Manhattan 10022

📞 (212) 751-0011

🌐 baumanrarebooks.com

$ Free admission (but you may succumb to a first-edition purchase)

🕐 Monday–Saturday, 10 a.m.–6 p.m.

🚌 **By subway:** E to Fifth Avenue/53rd Street; 6 to 51st Street.
By bus: M1, 2, 3, or 4 to 50th Street; M50 or 27 to Madison Avenue.

peaceful place 11

BIBLICAL GARDEN, CATHEDRAL CHURCH OF SAINT JOHN THE DIVINE

Upper West Side, Northern Manhattan

CATEGORY ⌣ spiritual enclaves ✪ ✪ ✪

*M*ost visitors stop inside the cathedral and fail to notice the small, secluded garden adjoining it. This vest-pocket park is preferred by neighborhood residents, who favor its solitude over the busier and noisier Morningside Park, a few blocks away, which is populated by dog walkers, preschoolers, skateboarders, and basketball players. Find the little garden by walking east along the southern edge of the cathedral to the garden. My favorite spots are by any one of the three gazebos. There, your senses can revel in the flowers' heady fragrance and the birds' twitters.

⌣ essentials

◪ 1047 Amsterdam Avenue (at 111th Street), Manhattan 10025

✆ (212) 316-7540

✈ stjohndivine.org

$ Free admission

☼ Open daily, sunrise to sunset.

🚌 **By subway:** 1 to 110th Street/Cathedral Parkway or 116th Street.
By bus: M104, 7, or 4 to Broadway/112th Street; M11 to Amsterdam Avenue/112th Street.

peaceful place 12

BIG CITY FISHING, PIER 84, HUDSON RIVER PARK
Midtown Manhattan

CATEGORY ⌣ outdoor habitats ✪

*A*nyone who fishes knows that the solitude and repose of casting, reeling, and waiting are at least as important as actually catching something. Anglers with their own gear can be found just about anywhere along New York City's shores, but at this pier, you can borrow gear from staffers and volunteers of the Hudson River Trust. You may also take free lessons on fishing and on the ecology and environment of the Hudson River Park's Estuarine Sanctuary. This public space is part of the Hudson River Park, which is managed by both the city and the state. In case you didn't know, the lower half of the mighty Hudson River isn't a freshwater river at all—it's a saltwater estuary with a tidal flow governed by the moon and the Atlantic Ocean. That's why Henry Hudson thought he had found the shortcut to the Far East in 1609, when this part of the world was truly secluded. Pier 84 is right next to the Intrepid Sea, Air & Space Museum, which is a World War II aircraft carrier, and even if you don't fish, it's well worth walking the length of the pier for a ground-level view of this magnificent ship.

⌣ essentials

≡˙   West 44th and West 43rd streets at the Hudson River; Manhattan 10036

☏   (212) 627-2020

🌐   hudsonriverpark.org/education/big_city_fishing.asp

$ Free admission, free instruction, and free use of all fishing supplies, including rods, reels, and bait. Supplies are provided on a first-come, first-served basis, with a half-hour limit on weekends.

🕐 Saturday–Sunday from Memorial Day to November 1 (weather permitting), 10:30 a.m.–5 p.m.

🚌 **By subway:** 1, 2, 3, 7, or S to Times Square; A, C, or E to 42nd Street.
By bus: M42 to the Hudson River.

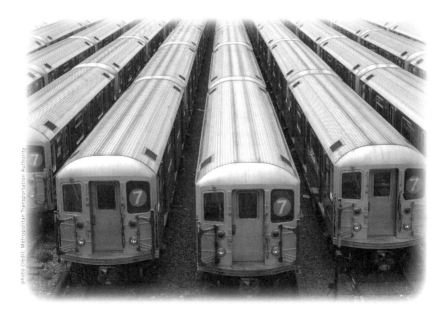

photo credit: Metropolitan Transportation Authority

New York City's subways and buses deliver you to peaceful spots.

peaceful place 13

BOATHOUSE, PROSPECT PARK
Park Slope, Brooklyn

CATEGORY ⌁ parks & gardens ✪ ✪ ✪

rand Army Plaza is Prospect Park's busy, throbbing heart, which makes the Beaux Arts Boathouse its brain. This is where you'll find the park visitor center, the Audubon Center with interactive exhibits on the area's wildlife and ecology, and Audubon guides and Urban Park Rangers who lead educational tours of the trails out back. The scenic guided boat ride on Prospect Park Lake that begins here is a relaxing escape, except on weekends. In keeping with the environmental mission of the park, you'll ride on a zero-emission electric boat with the added bonus of it being muffled enough to let you hear the fluttering feathers of the shorebirds you'll pass. Or, rent a pedal boat at adjoining Wollman Rink and get some exercise while you get close to the birds.

⌁ essentials

🖃   Flatbush and Ocean avenues to Prospect Park Southwest, between Parkside Avenue and Prospect Park West; Brooklyn 11215

📞   (718) 287-3400   🌐   prospectpark.org

$ Free admission. Electric boat is $8 for age 13 and up; $4 for children ages 4 to 12; free for children age 3 and under. $16.33 for pedal boats.

🕓   Open daily, sunrise to midnight. Electric boats: April–September, Thursday–Sunday, 12:30 p.m.–4:30 p.m. October: Saturday–Sunday, 12:30 p.m.–4:30 p.m. Pedal boats: May to mid-October, weather permitting.

🚌   By subway: S or B to Prospect Park; Q to Prospect Park or Parkside Avenue; 2 or 3 to Eastern Parkway. By bus: B69 or B75 to Prospect Park West and 9th Street; B68 to Prospect Park West and 15th Street.

peaceful place 14

BONNIE SLOTNICK COOKBOOKS
Greenwich Village, Lower Manhattan

CATEGORY ⌣ shops & services ✪ ✪

*R*elax at this delicious place with written words from some of the world's top chefs and restaurants. The shelves of this food-topic-only bookstore are crammed to the ceiling with everything from 18th-century recipe books to more current titles, plus antique kitchen tools and gadgets. There's something comforting about the happy clutter, which reminds me of a family kitchen at the center of the holidays, even without the aroma of mom's memorable apple pie baking in the oven. And the owner is almost always on hand to chat about food or share recipes.

⌣ essentials

⌐	163 West 10th Street (at Seventh Avenue South), Manhattan 10014
✆	(212) 989-8962
🌐	bonnieslotnickcookbooks.com
$	Free admission
🕐	Open 1 p.m.–7 p.m. six days a week, but the closed day varies, so phone first.
🚍	**By subway:** 1 to Christopher Street/Sheridan Square; A, B, C, D, E, or F to West 4th Street.

peaceful place 15

BOOKMARKS LOUNGE, LIBRARY HOTEL
Grand Central Station area, Midtown Manhattan

CATEGORY ↩ quiet tables ✪ ✪

*O*f course it is a cliché, but few things evoke more peacefulness than curling up in front of a soothing fire with a good book. All the better to do so at Bookmarks, the 14th-floor rooftop lounge of this charmingly themed luxury hotel. At the Bookmarks bar, you will enjoy one of the few working public fireplaces in Manhattan. Books and inviting chairs and sofas are placed comfortably about. Even the cocktail names have literary references and puns, such as The Hemingway and the Tequila Mockingbird. You will note, however, that Bookmarks' menu—and the fireplace—compete with the views from the 360-degree wraparound terrace. Plan your visit for the lounge's 4 p.m. opening, before the after-work and after-sightseeing crowd arrives to interrupt your solitude.

↩ essentials

✉	299 Madison Avenue (at 41st Street), Manhattan 10017
☎	(212) 983-4500
🌐	libraryhotel.com or hospitalityholdings.com
$	Free admission; drink prices are about $12 to $15
🕐	Monday–Saturday, 4 p.m.–midnight
🚌	**By subway:** 4, 5, 6, 7, or S to 42nd Street/Grand Central. **By bus:** M1, 2, 3, or 4 on Madison and Fifth avenues; M42 to 104th to 137th Street.

peaceful place 16

BROOKLYN BOTANIC GARDEN
Park Slope, Brooklyn
CATEGORY ✥ parks & gardens ✪ ✪ ✪

*T*ake your pick of venues amid this 52-acre oasis of green serenity with two-dozen specialty gardens. The Rose Garden alone is planted with some 1,200 varieties. I love spring, when the azalea, wisteria, and lilacs are in bloom. Also in spring, don't miss the Cherry Walk and Cherry Esplanade, a long, broad lawn bordered with double rows of trees sporting tiny pink and white blossoms. I like to sit on a bench just outside the esplanade, at a point where the trees seem to melt into the horizon. If it starts to get crowded, I escape to the Native Flora Garden, where the wood-chip trail past

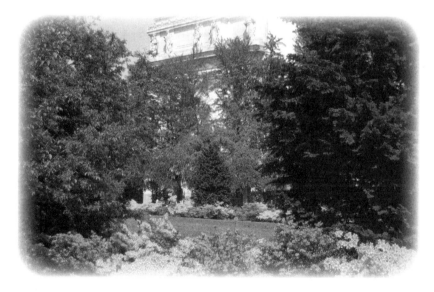

Brooklyn Botanic Garden

delicate ferns and massive oaks makes me forget that I am actually in New York City. And you can completely forget the 21st century in the cottage-style Shakespeare Garden, abloom with nearly 100 plants and flowers mentioned in the master's plays.

❣ essentials

📧 900 Washington Avenue, Brooklyn 11225 (Entrances are on Eastern Parkway adjoining the Brooklyn Museum; Flatbush Avenue at Empire Boulevard; and Washington Avenue.)

📞 (718) 623-7200

🌐 bbg.org

$ Adults $8; seniors and students $4; free for members and children under age 12; free for seniors on Fridays; free on Tuesdays, Saturdays 10–noon, and Monday–Friday mid-November to February

🕐 Mid-March to October: Tuesday–Friday, 8 a.m.–6 p.m.; Saturday–Sunday and some holiday Mondays, 10 a.m.–6 p.m. November to mid-March: Tuesday–Friday, 8 a.m.–4:30 p.m. and Saturday–Sunday and some holiday Mondays, 10 a.m.–4:30 p.m.

🚌 **By subway:** 2 or 3 to Eastern Parkway; B, Q, or S to Prospect Park.
By bus: B71 to the museum; B48 to Franklin Avenue and Eastern Parkway.

peaceful place 17

BROOKLYN BRIDGE PARK
Brooklyn Heights, Brooklyn
CATEGORY ↵ scenic vistas ✪ ✪ ✪

*P*ark entrances at Old Fulton Street and Atlantic Avenue, plus Piers 1 and 6 —altogether the first sections of this long-planned 85-acre park—opened in 2009. Each pier is the size of several city blocks and is beautifully landscaped with water gardens and mixed-use bike and skating paths. But the real draws for me are the drop-dead views of Lower Manhattan from the wide esplanade. With links to the Empire-Fulton Ferry State Park, this site adds up to mile-plus drink-of-water views from south of the Brooklyn Bridge to just north of the Manhattan Bridge. Did I mention the sunsets? When completed in 2012, there are to be several miles of floating paths, sandy beaches, coves and canals, and kayak and canoe paddling areas in restored wetlands and tidal inlets. This is a brilliant new use for abandoned, rotting piers and buildings that's been more than a decade in the planning. It makes me feel peaceful just to think about the green revolution at this site.

↵ essentials

🖃 One Main Street, Atlantic Avenue to Jay Street, East Rive; Brooklyn 11201

☏ (718) 802-0603   🌐 brooklynbridgepark.org and brooklynbridgeparknyc.org

$ Free admission   🕙 Open daily, 6 a.m.–1 a.m.

🚌 **By subway:** A or C to High Street; 2 or 3 to Clark Street; F to York Street.
By bus: B25 to Fulton Ferry Landing. From Memorial Day to Labor Day, New York Water Taxi (nywatertaxi.com) commutes between Lower Manhattan and the park.

BROOKLYN HEIGHTS ESPLANADE
Brooklyn Heights, Brooklyn
CATEGORY ↵ scenic vistas ✪ ✪ ✪

*B*e forewarned: Nobody in Brooklyn calls this by its official name. If you ask a passerby which way to the esplanade, you'll get a blank look or a shrug. That's because everybody knows it simply as the promenade. This magnificent esplanade-cum-promenade offers a picture-postcard view of the Brooklyn Bridge, of course, across to Lower Manhattan. As a bonus, it frames glimpses of the Statue of Liberty to the south, the Brooklyn Bridge, Empire State and Chrysler buildings to the north, and the Staten Island Ferry in between. Stay back from the wrought-iron fence if you have vertigo: The Brooklyn-Queens Expressway runs just below, and one lane of the highway traffic is visible if you look over the railing. Joggers, dog walkers, and baby strollers dominate the promenade, but the uneven flagstones are not user-friendly to hotshot skateboarders. Head for the benches that line the blocks of the promenade. They offer an ideal spot to read a book or enjoy a picnic lunch—perhaps the one you assembled on Atlantic Avenue (see page 12). While the afternoon sun warms your face, inhale both the view and the hint of salt air that drifts in from the Atlantic Ocean when the wind is right.

My own favorite time is just before sunset, when there's a golden glow on the mirrored facades of Lower Manhattan's skyscrapers, and the light dances through the cobweblike support wires of the Brooklyn Bridge, creating wonderfully eerie patterns of color and shadow. It should not be a surprise that the promenade is most crowded on weekends in warm weather, since—after all—this is Brooklyn's front yard. But you know what to do—just savor your time during the week.

✧ essentials

✉ Remsen Street to Orange Street along the East River; Brooklyn 11201

☎ (718) 802-3846   🌐 visitbrooklyn.org

$ Free admission   🕐 Open daily, 24 hours

🚌 **By subway:** 2, 3, M, or R to Court Street; A, C, or F to Jay Street/Borough Hall.

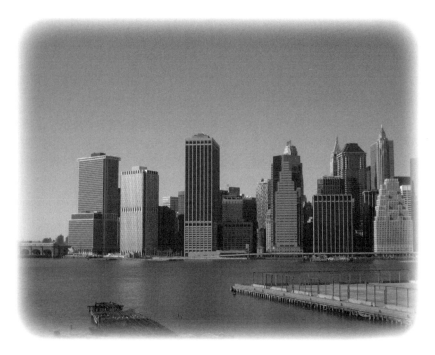

City view from Brooklyn Heights Esplanade

peaceful place 19

BROOKLYN HEIGHTS SELF-GUIDED WALKING TOUR
Brooklyn Heights, Brooklyn

CATEGORY ↵ enchanting walks ✪ ✪

*B*lock after block of this tidy residential neighborhood is lined with lovely redbrick and stone Victorian town houses. Small gardens and front steps bookended by filigreed wrought-iron balustrades complete the setting. Larger apartment buildings—some of them former one-family mansions—are decorated with gargoyles and carved stone froufrous. Even the street names speak to the past and will lure you to meander: Cranberry, Pineapple, and Willow; Joralemon, Pierrepont, and Montague; and my favorite, Love Lane. I like to stop in front of 24 Middagh Street to gaze at a wooden house built in 1824. It's in better shape than some New York City skyscrapers from the 1950s. Another favorite is the fine Greek Revival mansion at 70 Willow Street, where Truman Capote lived in 1958 when he wrote *Breakfast at Tiffany's*.

Unfortunately, escalating rents have forced out most of the tiny boutiques, independent bookstores, and art galleries that used to line Montague Street, the Heights' main thoroughfare, and make it such a pleasant stroll. Now, it's just bank branch after bank branch and clothing chain after clothing chain—a busy commercial street to walk through quickly to get to the Brooklyn Heights Esplanade (see page 26) and the picturesque side streets.

essentials

State Street to Cadman Plaza, Brooklyn-Queens Expressway to East River; Brooklyn 11201

(718) 802-3846 $ Free admission

galttech.com/research/travel/brooklyn-heights-promenade-walking-tour.php for a map for the self-guided walking tour

Open daily

By subway: 2, 3, M, or R to Court Street; 4, 5, A, C, or F to Jay Street/Borough Hall.

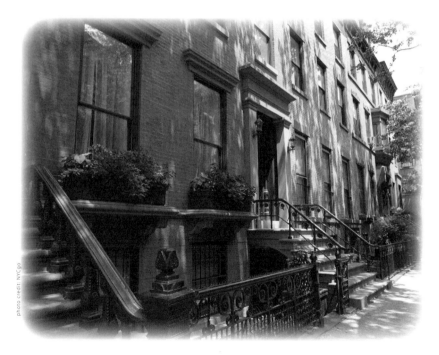

photo credit: NYCgo

Shady porches in Brooklyn Heights

peaceful place 20

BROOKLYN HISTORICAL SOCIETY

Brooklyn Heights, Brooklyn

CATEGORY ↙ reading rooms ✪ ✪

his landmark four-story Queen Anne–style building dates from 1881 and offers an elegant escape on a scale as grand as the interior's sweeping staircase. The library is distinguished with carved black ash wainscoting that falls shoulder high on five-foot-one me. It seems a very dignified place for an absorbing history lesson. Ornamenting the walls are portraits of significant Revolutionary Era and Victorian Brooklynites, including Philip Livingston, who helped draft and sign the Declaration of Independence. He lived a couple of blocks away, on Hicks Street, where General George Washington stayed after the Battle of Brooklyn.

Ever-changing exhibits lead you through Brooklyn's history—from Dutch Colonial times to the modern disappearance of Montague Street storefronts. The absolute best thing about this facility, though, is its two-story library, which would feel right at home in a Charles Dickens or Emily Brontë novel. Here you can relish the black ash bookcases and carved balcony, the ladders for reaching books on the upper shelves, and the reading tables with apothecary-style lampshade lights. The Othmer Library and Archives is not a lending library, but a research facility for genealogy and history about Brooklyn and Long Island. It's also a great place to park yourself in another century. With or without a book.

⌣ essentials

☑ 128 Pierrepont Street (at Clinton Street), Brooklyn 11201

📞 (718) 222-4111

🌐 brooklynhistory.org

$ Adults $6; seniors and students $4; free for children under age 12

🕐   Wednesday–Friday, noon–5 p.m.; Saturday, 10 a.m.–5 p.m.; Sunday, noon–5 p.m.
    (library closed Sundays).

🚍 **By subway:** M or R to Court Street; 2, 3, 4, or 5 to Borough Hall;
    A, C, or F to Jay Street/Borough Hall.
    By bus: B38, 52, 25, 26, or 41 to Montague/Court Street; B67 or 65 to Jay Street.

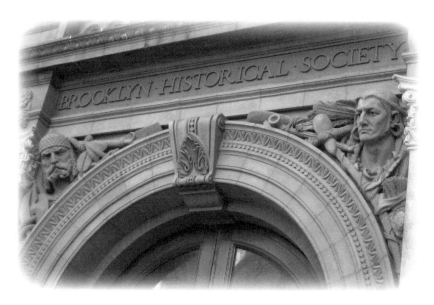

The Brooklyn Historical Society's 1881 building

peaceful place 21

BROOKLYN MUSEUM
Park Slope, Brooklyn

CATEGORY ↙ museums & galleries ✪ ✪

*A*nywhere else on earth, this would be a world-class museum, but this Beaux Arts gem is the second-place stepsister to the better-known Metropolitan Museum of Art in Manhattan. This works to the advantage of tranquility seekers, since this museum is rarely crowded. It's easy to find an isolated spot even when school groups are in attendance. I usually head straight for the sprawling Egypt wing on the third floor to contemplate the still-vibrant decorations on the sarcophagi and lifelike statues, and I wonder if anything we create today will still be admired 3,000 years from now. Wednesdays and Thursdays are the calmest days to visit.

essentials

200 Eastern Parkway, Brooklyn 11238

(718) 638-5000   brooklynmuseum.org

$ Suggested contribution: adults $10; seniors and students $6; free for members and children under age 12 accompanied by a paying adult.

Wednesday–Friday, 10 a.m.–5 p.m.; Saturday–Sunday, 11 a.m.–6 p.m. and to 11 p.m. on the first Saturday of each month.

By subway: 2 or 3 to Eastern Parkway.
By bus: B71 to museum; B48 to Franklin Avenue and Eastern Parkway.

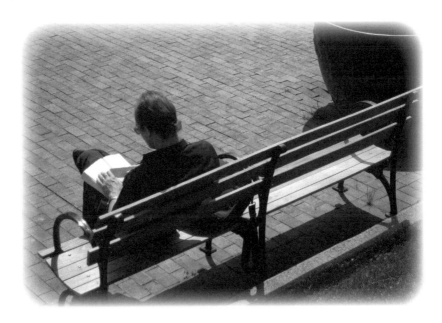

Outside Brooklyn Museum

peaceful place 22

BROOKVILLE PARK
Rosedale, Queens

CATEGORY ⌣ outdoor habitats ✪ ✪

*A*t only 90 acres, Brookville is small by Queens standards, and that is just the start of its appeal. For me, the best parts are the small pond and the walking and biking trail. The trail winds along the brook for which the park is named and which drains into nearby Jamaica Bay. The occasional pheasant or hawk is not scared away by the low-flying jets soaring into or out of JFK's airway, just beyond the park. There's actually a restful rhythm to the clocklike regularity of the jets. They tend to trigger in me the escapist nonsense of recognizing airline logos. That reminds me of the "red car, green car" and license plate games I played as a child on family road trips, long before the advent of backseat entertainment screens and live satellite TV. Those thoughts alone are peaceful.

⌣ essentials

🖃	149th Avenue to South Conduit Avenue, between Brookville Boulevard and 232nd Street; Queens 11422
☏	(212) 639-9675
🌐	nycgovparks.org/parks/Q008
$	Free admission
🕑	Open daily, 7 a.m.–9 p.m.
🚋	**By rail/subway:** Take the Long Island Rail Road to Rosedale Station, and walk about 10 minutes to 233rd Street to the park entrance.

peaceful place 23

BRYANT PARK
Midtown Manhattan

CATEGORY ↝ parks & gardens ✪ ✪

One block from Times Square, you will find one of the most interesting parks in the city, with flagstone walkways and a small carousel. The carousel is my favorite. There's no calliope music, but the movement of its shapes and colors mesmerizes me. In winter, part of the huge open lawn is covered by an ice-skating rink. In warm weather, workers from nearby offices occupy the wrought-iron chairs and tables for lunchtime respites. Bryant Park also lures professionals hanging out between appointments, thumbing furiously on their BlackBerrys or iPhones.

The park's checkered history ranges from its use as a potter's field in the early 1800s, when this was the northern edge of Manhattan, to its selection as the site of the 1853 World's Fair. A century later, it became a dangerous, crime-infested place to avoid. The park has since been re-invented, re-seeded, and re-planted into a bright and safe Midtown greenway, uncrowded except for weekday lunchtimes. Another time you won't find tranquility here is when the annual Fashion Week designer shows take over the area of the park closest to Sixth Avenue. Otherwise, my favorite period to visit is Tuesday or Thursday mornings for the free tai chi class—May to mid-October, 7:30 a.m.; (212) 221-6110, chutaichi.com.

↝ essentials

📧 Fifth and Sixth Avenue between 40th and 42nd streets, Manhattan 10036

📞 (212) 768-4242

🌐 nycgovparks.org/parks/bryantpark or bryantpark.org

$ Free admission

🕐   Open daily. January–March: 7 a.m.–7 p.m.; to 10 p.m. in January while pond is open; to 8 p.m. after Daylight Saving Time begins. April, November, and December: 7 a.m.–10 p.m. May–September: 7 a.m.–11 p.m. October: 7 a.m.–8 p.m.

🚌   **By subway:** 1, 2, or 3 to Times Square; F, B, or D to 42nd Street/Bryant Park; 7 to Fifth Avenue.
     By bus: M42 or 104 to Sixth Avenue; M4, 5, 6, or 7 to 42nd Street.

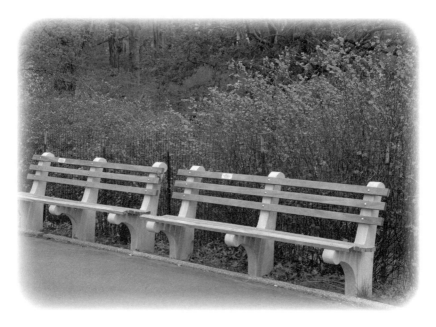

Have a seat on one of New York City's many park benches.

peaceful place 24

CADMAN PLAZA PARK
Brooklyn Heights, Brooklyn

CATEGORY ᴗ parks & gardens ✪

nfolding for several blocks, this open green space splits the cluster of Brooklyn's official buildings from Brooklyn Heights. Despite being surrounded on all sides by noisy bus and car traffic, it attracts joggers to its long, straight sidewalks and paths; touch football and soccer players and local families flock to its greens on weekends. So the best time for solitude here is weekdays when the kids are in school and the office workers are at their desks. Watch for peregrine falcons, or visit the park's World War II memorial.

ᴗ essentials

☰ Tillary to Prospect streets, between Cadman Plaza East (Washington Street) and Cadman Plaza West (Court Street); Brooklyn 11201

☎ (212) 639-9675

🌐 nycgovparks.org/parks/cadmanplazapark

$ Free admission

🕐 Open daily, 6 a.m.–1 a.m.

🚇 **By subway:** 2 or 3, M or R to Court Street; A, C, or F to Jay Street/Borough Hall.

peaceful place 25

CAFÉ SFA, SAKS FIFTH AVENUE
Midtown Manhattan

CATEGORY ⌣ quiet tables ✪ ✪

*N*ormally, I wouldn't recommend a restaurant or cafe inside a department store, but this one is exceptional—not so much for its food or decor, but for the view. For years, Saks Fifth Avenue used this space overlooking its namesake avenue as a stockroom area. Wisely, somebody a few years ago realized that it wasn't smart to allocate prime real estate that way and turned this fourth-floor spot into one of the best views in town, directly across Fifth Avenue from the Channel Gardens and Rockefeller Plaza. It's a great place to observe the annual holiday tree. Skip lunchtime, when it's crowded with shoppers hungry for the latest fashions, and opt instead for afternoon tea starting at 3 p.m., when the afternoon light throws pleasant shadows across the scene.

⌣ essentials

✉	611 Fifth Avenue inside Saks Fifth Avenue (at 49th and 50th streets), Manhattan 10022
✆	(212) 940-4080 🌐 saksfifthavenue.com
$	Free admission; cost varies by menu item, $9 to $28
🕐	Monday–Saturday, 11 a.m.–5 p.m.; Sunday, noon–5 p.m.
🚌	**By subway:** B, D, or F to 47th-50th Street; N, R, or W to 49th Street. **By bus:** M1, 2, 3, 4, 5, 6, or 7 to 50th Street; M27 or 50 to Fifth Avenue; M6 to 51st Street.

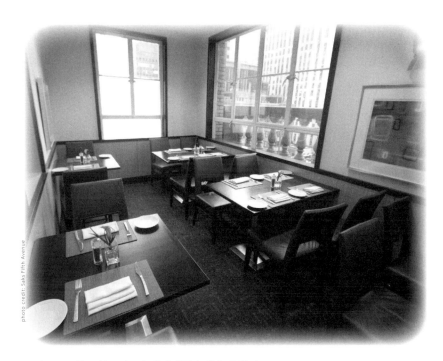

photo credit: Saks Fifth Avenue

Corner table with a view in Café SFA in Saks Fifth Avenue

peaceful place 26

CAMPBELL APARTMENT
Grand Central Station, Midtown Manhattan

CATEGORY ↩ quiet tables ✪

*J*ust steps from the bustle of the Grand Central Terminal concourse and its platforms sits an oasis of carved-wood paneled walls, an ornate carved ceiling, expansive stained glass windows, a grand stone fireplace, Oriental carpets, and welcoming sofas and chairs. The scene reminds me of a room in a Vanderbilt mansion or in the castle of a European noble, but this escape is inside the station. It's one of those word-of-mouth spots that have a following, but if you come in mid-afternoon—before the after-work arrival of those in the know—you can indulge in a blissfully quiet interlude. The Campbell Apartment was the private office of John W. Campbell, a millionaire who served on the board of the New York Central Railroad and who died in 1957. Now it beckons you for a very hospitable cocktail.

↩ essentials

≡ 15 Vanderbilt Avenue (between 42nd and 43rd streets), inside Grand Central Terminal; Manhattan 10017

☎ (212) 953-0409   ☝ hospitalityholdings.com

$ Free admission; drink prices are about $13 to $16 (dress code applies)

🕐 Monday–Thursday, noon–1 a.m.; Friday, noon–2 a.m.; Saturday, 3 p.m.–2 a.m.; Sunday, 3 p.m.–11 p.m.

🚌 **By subway:** 4, 5, 6, 7, or S to 42nd Street/Grand Central.
By bus: M42 or 104 to Vanderbilt Avenue; M1, 2, 3, 4, 101, 102, or 103 to 42nd Street.

peaceful place 27

CANARSIE PIER, GATEWAY NATIONAL RECREATION AREA

Brooklyn

CATEGORY ↲ outdoor habitats ✪

*P*ardon my pun, but it's no fluke that this 600-foot pier is so popular with anglers: It has some of the best fishing for fluke, bluefish, and other species in Jamaica Bay. Whether you cast a line or not, the pier extends a wonderfully soothing setting for reeling in views of the protected shoreline and salt marshes surrounding it. And you know you can count on fishermen to keep quiet. So find your spot either to hook a few or just to dangle your feet over the pier and re-create a Huckleberry Finn experience far from the Mississippi. In the summer, the National Park Service offers a free kayak program on Sundays, 10 a.m.–2 p.m., at the end of the pier; no reservations required. Group kayaking is held on Fridays; and on Mondays, different locations and skill levels are highlighted. Both are offered in season, are free, and are by reservation only.

↲ essentials

⊟ Canarsie Pier (at Shore and Rockaway parkways), Brooklyn 11236

✆ (718) 763-2202

➍ nyharborparks.org/visit/capi.html

$ Free admission

🕔 Open daily, 5 a.m.–2 a.m.

🚌 **By subway and bus:** L to Rockaway Peninsula and transfer to bus B42 to the pier.

peaceful place 28

CATHEDRAL CHURCH OF SAINT JOHN THE DIVINE
Upper West Side, Northern Manhattan

CATEGORY ↶ spiritual enclaves ✪ ✪ ✪

*T*he monumental Gothic features of this landmark are a given, and they always provide soulful relief. For me, the most soothing experience comes when sunlight pours through the extraordinary stained-glass windows. The best time to visit is in the morning, until about noon, for the window above the high altar, and mid-afternoon for the stained glass in the nave. The cathedral also is well known for its concerts. My choice is the annual Paul Winter Consort's Summer Solstice program. It begins in the dark, at 4:30 a.m., as if to welcome the first day of summer, and the music continues as the dawn lights the stained-glass jewels. It is mesmerizing. Another favorite is the cathedral's free organ recital every Monday at 1 p.m. The presentation is called an organ demonstration, but it is truly well-played music for enchanted listeners.

↶ essentials

▤   1047 Amsterdam Avenue (at 112th Street), Manhattan 10025

✆   (212) 316-7540

🌐   stjohndivine.org

$ Free admission; tours $5; cost varies for concerts

🕐 Monday–Saturday, 7 a.m.–6 p.m.; Sunday, 7 a.m.–7 p.m. Tours: Tuesday–Saturday, 11 a.m. and 1 p.m.; Sunday, 2 p.m.

🚌 **By subway:** 1 or C to 110th Street/Cathedral Parkway or 116th Street.
By bus: M104, 7, 11, or 60 to Broadway/112th Street; M11 or 4 to Amsterdam Avenue/112th Street.

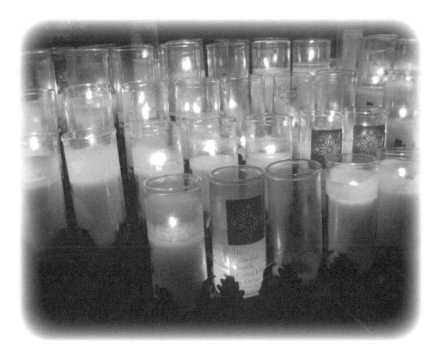

Devotional candles burning at Cathedral Church of Saint John the Divine

peaceful place 29

CELEBRITY PATH, BROOKLYN BOTANIC GARDEN
Park Slope, Brooklyn

CATEGORY ⌇ enchanting walks ✪ ✪

*J*ust beyond the popular Japanese Hill-and-Pond Garden, a shaded little path looks as if it doesn't lead anywhere. That is exactly why it is one of the least-used and therefore most secluded spots in this park. The path is paved with flagstones naming famous Brooklynites—from the Roebelings, who built the Brooklyn Bridge, to singer Barbra Streisand and composer George Gershwin. Follow it to the end, where you will be rewarded by the charm of a small amphitheater with curved, terraced stone benches. I like to sit near the top, for a capsule view of the Japanese garden's pond and its magnificent red and black Torii arch in dappled sunlight through the trees.

⌇ essentials

🖃   900 Washington Avenue, Brooklyn 11225 (Entrances are on Eastern Parkway adjoining the Brooklyn Museum; Flatbush Avenue at Empire Boulevard; and Washington Avenue.)

𝒞   (718) 623-7200   🌐 bbg.org

$ Adults $8; seniors and students $4; free for members and children under age 12; free for seniors on Fridays; free on Tuesdays, Saturdays 10–noon, and Monday–Friday mid-November to February

🕐   Mid-March to October: Tuesday–Friday, 8 a.m.–6 p.m.; Saturday–Sunday and some holiday Mondays, 10 a.m.–6 p.m. November to mid-March: Tuesday–Friday, 8 a.m.–4:30 p.m.; Saturday–Sunday and some holiday Mondays, 10 a.m.–4:30 p.m.

🚉   **By subway:** 2 or 3 to Eastern Parkway; B, Q, or S to Prospect Park.
By bus: B71 to the museum; B48 to Franklin Avenue and Eastern Parkway.

peaceful place 30

CHANNEL GARDENS, ROCKEFELLER CENTER
Midtown Manhattan

CATEGORY ⌣ urban surprises ✪

he gardens create a broad promenade that separates Rockefeller Center's French Building from the British Empire Building, much as the English Channel separates the two countries—hence its name. Displays rotate from fanciful topiaries to ethereal orchids, depending on the season, and during the holidays, the gardens are decked out in lights to frame the iconic Rockefeller Center Christmas tree on the Rockefeller Plaza side of the famous ice-skating rink. During peak tourist seasons (Thanksgiving to New Year's and summer), it can be pretty crowded until dinnertime, but other times you will find lots of places to perch on benches and soak up the sunshine. If you pick a bench facing west, you'll see the fluttering flags of United Nations member countries; on benches facing east you can contemplate the shadows dancing around the towering spires of St. Patrick's Cathedral.

⌣ essentials

🖃	Between 49th and 50th streets, off Fifth Avenue, Manhattan 10111
☎	(212) 332-6868
🌐	rockefellercenter.com
$	Free admission
🕐	Open daily, 24 hours
🚌	**By subway:** B, D, or F to 47th-50th Street; N, R, or W to 49th Street. **By bus:** M1, 2, 3, 4, 5, 6, or 7 to 50th Street; M27 or 50 to Fifth Avenue; M6 to 51st Street.

peaceful place 31

CHARTWELL BOOKSELLERS
Midtown Manhattan

CATEGORY ⌣ shops & services ✪ ✪

ecause I am a great fan of vintage and antique cars, this is my favorite place for a virtual ride. I like to cruise in low speed among the shelves of books about historic Porsches, Ferraris, Rolls-Royces, and such. But you don't have to share my automobile habit to want to come here. An antiquarian bookshop, Chartwell specializes in quite an assemblage of topics; among them is Winston Churchill. The shop is named after his home outside London, and elegant bronze and glass showcases hold Churchill memorabilia. Or perhaps your interests embrace baseball, military history, jazz history, and luscious photography books by such icons as nature specialist Ansel Adams and fashion's Richard Avedon. If so, this will become your haven, too.

⌣ essentials

≡	55 East 52nd Street (in the arcade of the Park Avenue Plaza Building), Manhattan 10055
☎	(212) 308-0643
⊕	chartwellbooksellers.com
$	Free admission
☒	Monday–Friday, 10 a.m.–6 p.m., and Saturdays in December
⛟	**By subway:** E or F to Fifth Avenue; 6 to 51st Street. **By bus:** M4 or 5 to 52nd Street; M50 to Madison or Lexington avenues.

peaceful place 32

CHELSEA COVE, HUDSON RIVER PARK
Lower Manhattan

CATEGORY ⌣ scenic vistas ✪ ✪

*W*hen fully completed, Piers 62, 63, and 64 are to include a large green lawn "bowl," a spectacular garden, and a landscape sculpture consisting of a boulder field, so it's easy to pick which type of solitude and inspiration fits your particular mood of the moment. The rebuilt Pier 62 already features a carousel and makes an ideal spot to sit and commune with memories of childhood. My vote for the best spot is at the end of the long, green Pier 64. It offers incredible views to the north and south, just past a grove of trees that lures you to investigate the farther reaches of this pier park. At press time, Pier 64 and its green embellishments were scheduled for completion by spring 2010.

⌣ essentials

▤	22nd Street to 25th Street at the Hudson River, Manhattan 10011
✆	(212) 627-2020
✈	hudsonriverpark.org
$	Free admission
◔	Open daily, 6 a.m.–1 a.m.
🚌	**By subway and bus:** 1, C, or E to 23rd Street, then the M23 or 14 bus to pier.

peaceful place 33

CHERRY WALK, RIVERSIDE PARK
Upper West Side, Northern and Upper Manhattan

CATEGORY ⌣ enchanting walks ✪

*V*isit in April, when hundreds of cherry trees bloom in pink and white glory. But everybody else knows this, too, and this picturesque walkway a few feet from the Hudson River stays popular all summer, especially on weekends. So I prefer it on a crisp autumn afternoon, or after the spring and summer crowds have gone home to make dinner and put the kids to bed. Then I can have the sunset over the Hudson all to myself. The walkway is unusual in that it changes from a flat and open space to a squeeze between boulders. Before you set out, be forewarned: Once you enter this stretch between the river and the West Side Highway, there is no exit until you reach the other end, one mile away. So, my other tip is this: Have a hearty lunch or brunch of smoky ribs and fixings at Dinosaur Bar-B-Que—646 West 131st Street, 10027, (212) 694-1777, dinosaurbarbque.com—and walk off the calories as you head south. For an alternative stroll lined with cherry trees and benches, follow the three-block stretch between 93rd and 96th streets.

⌣ essentials

☰ 100th Street to 125th Street along Hudson River (enter at Riverside Drive at 98th Street), Manhattan 10025 and 10027

✆ (212) 408-0264   ➤ nycgovparks.org/parks/riversidepark $ Free admission

⏱ Open daily, 6 a.m.–1 a.m., but not recommended after sunset

🚌 **By subway:** 1, 2, or 3 to 96th Street; 1 to 125th Street.
By bus: M104 to 98th or 125th streets; M96 or Bx15 to Riverside Drive.

peaceful place 34

CHESS SHOPS OF GREENWICH VILLAGE
Lower Manhattan
CATEGORY ⌣ shops & services ✪ ✪

*I*f deep concentration delivers you to a peaceful state, then these two Thompson Street shops, both of which have been in the neighborhood for over a decade, should be your next destination. If you like chess, that is, and if you like dueling chess shops. Quietly dueling, of course, since chess matches are by their nature quiet competitions for both players and onlookers. And watching is encouraged. Chess Forum sells rare chess sets, including one that features the super-rival New York Yankees and Boston Red Sox baseball teams. Village Chess Shop also sells chess sets, but it seems to have more people playing chess there. Village Chess Shop has the added attraction of a sound system that serenades you with classical music in the background. You can also play live chess here for $2.50 an hour—not bad prices in this not-exactly-low-rent neighborhood.

⌣ essentials

- 219 and 230 Thompson Street, respectively, Manhattan 10012
- Chess Forum: (212) 475-2369; Village Chess Shop: (212) 475-9580
- chessforum.com; chess-shop.com $ Free admission; $2.50 per hour to play chess
- Open daily, 11 a.m.–midnight
- **By subway:** F, A, C, E, B, or D to West Fourth Street (Waverly Place exit); 2 or 3 to 14th Street; 1 to Christopher Street.

peaceful place 35

CITY HALL PARK
Lower Manhattan

CATEGORY ↝ parks & gardens ✪

ntil 1699, this parcel was a communal pasture for livestock; then it became the site of a debtor's prison and public hangings. Today, it's a hideaway with Victorian-style lampposts, a large fountain, and lush plantings, so there's a distinct historic feel, which is appropriate considering its municipal neighbor. There are plenty of spots to sit, except during midday when it's crowded with lunch-bag office workers. Avoid late afternoon, too, since the park is located where several major streets converge for the Brooklyn Bridge entrance, and horn-honking is endemic. Once you have achieved a state of bliss, you can take your new attitude just across from the park and over to J&R [(800) 806-1115, jr.com], one of the city's top electronics, computer, and photographic emporiums. It may be far from peaceful, since it's almost always jammed with shoppers checking out the latest gear at bargain prices, but the discounts provide reassurance to your bank account.

↝ essentials

▭   Broadway to Park Row at Chambers Street, Manhattan 10007

☎ (212) 639-9675   🌐 nycgovparks.org/parks/cityhallpark

$ Free admission   🕐 Open daily, 6 a.m.–1 a.m.

🚇 **By subway:** 4, 5, or 6 to Brooklyn Bridge/City Hall; 2 or 3 to Park Row; R or W to City Hall; J or M to Fulton Street.
By bus: M1 or 22 to Park Row or Chambers Street.

peaceful place 36

CLOISTERS, FORT TRYON PARK
Washington Heights, Northern Manhattan

CATEGORY ↙ museums & galleries ✪ ✪ ✪

Perched like a stone tiara atop one of the tallest hills of Manhattan, located in Fort Tryon Park, this is medieval Europe on the Hudson. Here for viewing are enough stained glass, stone statues, silver chalices, and illuminated manuscripts from the 12th to the 16th centuries to soothe even the most troubled soul. The site contains five French and Spanish cloisters reassembled here like a monumental jigsaw puzzle. The John D. Rockefeller Jr. family, which wanted a proper setting for its world-famous 15th-century Unicorn Tapestries, financed the project in the 1930s. These treasures are showcased in their own darkened room. Tranquility also reigns elsewhere in this northern outpost of the Metropolitan Museum of Art: Most visitors are plugged in to audio guides and therefore are not speaking, and when they do, it's in hushed tones.

After the room housing the seven gigantic tapestries, I have two other favorite spots to recommend. One, the West Terrace, lures me with its panoramic view across the Hudson River and along the downtown Manhattan skyline. To reach the West Terrace, go through the wooden door on the right side of the Pontaut Chapter House. My other favorite is the Cuxa Cloister, a colonnaded garden in the center of the complex. This respite is inviting almost year-round with its ever-changing plantings and, in warm weather, its fluttering hummingbirds are something to behold. Mornings are the best times to visit the Cloisters, but check the Web site and go whenever there is a concert featuring medieval and early Renaissance music, which seems particularly soothing on a cold winter day.

essentials

99 Margaret Corbin Drive, Fort Tryon Park, Manhattan 10040

(212) 923-3700   metmuseum.org/cloisters

$ Adults $20; seniors $15; students $10; free for members and children under age 12 accompanied by a paying adult. (Fees include same-day admission to the Metropolitan Museum of Art's main building on Fifth Avenue and 82nd Street.)

March–October: Tuesday–Sunday, 9:30 a.m.–5:15 p.m. November–February: 9:30 a.m.–4:45 p.m.

By subway: A to 190th Street, then take the elevator to Overlook Terrace, then take the M4 bus to last stop.

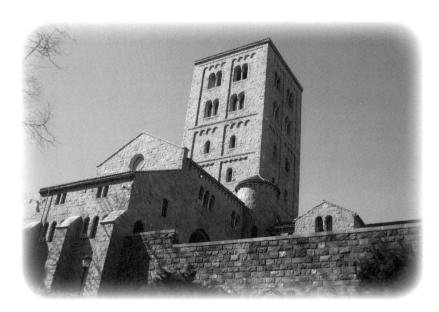

The Cloisters atop one of the tallest hills of Manhattan

COLUMBIA UNIVERSITY QUAD
Upper West Side, Northern Manhattan

CATEGORY ⌣ enchanting walks ✪

he formidable facade of the Low Memorial Library, completed in 1897, dominates the enormous, grassy quad. I like walking up the broad stone steps to watch the sunlight dance on the building's Beaux Arts features. Another pastime is to sit on one of the high steps to take in the ballet of movement when students change classes, or just to relax and catch up on reading. The building no longer serves as a library and instead houses the university's administrative offices. The visitor center, located in room 213 of the former library, offers brochures for self-guided walking tours, and I enjoy walking among the quad's historic buildings and imposing statues. Whenever I visit the campus, I always make a pilgrimage to Journalism Hall, built in 1912 with money donated by Joseph Pulitzer. Carry a couple of books or the day's newspaper, dress comfortably, and—depending on your age—it will be assumed you are either a grad student or a professor.

⌣ essentials

⌹ 116th Street and Broadway, Manhattan 10027

🕭 (212) 854-1754   🗱 columbia.edu

$ Free admission   🕧 Visitor center: Monday–Friday, 9 a.m.–5 p.m.

🚌 **By subway:** 1 to 116th Street.
By bus: M4, 7, 11, or 104 to 116th Street.

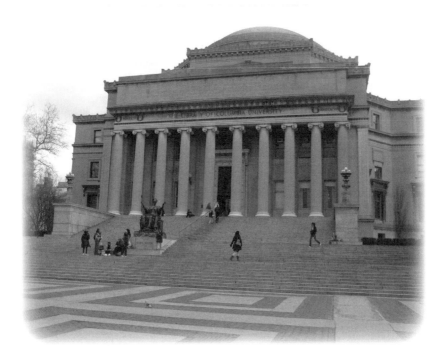

The Low Memorial Library at Columbia University Quad

peaceful place 38

CONSERVATORY GARDEN, CENTRAL PARK
Upper East Side, Upper Manhattan

CATEGORY ⌣ parks & gardens ✪ ✪ ✪

Welcome to one of Central Park's few official Quiet Zones, which you enter through an ornate two-story wrought-iron gate. Guarding the Vanderbilt Mansion almost a century ago, the massive portal today implies that something special still lies beyond its arch. And it does. While bike riding and skating are not allowed— good news for those looking for tranquility here—partaking of the many well-placed benches certainly is permitted. Scattered amid six acres of formal gardens in Italian, French, and English landscape styles, the seating invites you to hide out for a while and ignore the nearby bustle of Upper East Side traffic.

My favorite niche beckons beneath the Victorian wrought-iron pergola twined with wisteria. This offers a strategic vantage point for peering out to stepped ledges of flowering shrubs, which lead to the manicured lawn of the Italian garden. The garden, named for an 1898 glass conservatory that was demolished in the 1930s, remains idyllic anytime. Even when wedding couples commandeer some picture-perfect spots for their portraits, you'll simply want to smile.

⌣ essentials

▤	105th Street and Fifth Avenue, Manhattan 10029		
☏	(212) 310-6600	◉	centralparknyc.org
$	Free admission	◷	Open daily, 8 a.m. to sunset
▦	**By subway:** 2 or 3 to 110th Street. **By bus:** M1, 2, 3, 4, or 96 to 105th Street.		

peaceful place 39

DEAD HORSE BAY, GATEWAY NATIONAL RECREATION AREA

Flatbush, Brooklyn

CATEGORY ↝ outdoor habitats ✪ ✪

A trio of short trails fans out like a fleur-de-lis from a single entrance into the marshland. It begins a few hundred yards from the tollbooths of the Gil Hodges Memorial Bridge, which links Brooklyn and Queens across Jamaica Bay. All three trails lead to different parts of the bay and inlet, with grassy paths that turn into sandy strips close to water's edge. And with all three, as your walk approaches the shoreline, the tall inland shade trees give way to scrub pine and grasses. My favorite trail in this part of the Gateway National Recreation Area is the one on the left. It leads to a little beach with a view across the inlet to the residential community of Breezy Point. Except for the recognizable bridge, you could be on Nantucket or Block Island. You can walk all three trails at a leisurely pace inside of an hour—longer if you stop to watch the hawks, jackrabbits, seabirds, and the occasional passing pleasure boat. There are better-known and longer nature trails elsewhere in the sprawling park, but their near anonymity is what makes these three so peaceful, even on a summer weekend. The trail entrance is across the road from the National Park Service ranger station at Floyd Bennett Field, where you can pick up a trail map.

↝ essentials

▭ 50 Aviation Road, Brooklyn 11234

✆ (718) 338-3799   🌐 nps.gov/gate $ Free admission

🕐 National Park Service ranger station: Friday–Tuesday, 9 a.m.–5 p.m. Trails: open daily, sunrise to sunset.

🚇 **By subway and bus:** 2 to Flatbush Avenue or A to Rockaway Park/Beach 116th Street, then bus Q35 to the ranger station.

peaceful place 40

DYCKMAN FARMHOUSE MUSEUM
Northern Manhattan

CATEGORY ↶ historic sites ✪ ✪

I grew up near the Dyckman Farmhouse and went to school across the street. When weather permitted, I did my homework amid its sheltering trees and colorful flowers and called it my secret garden. I am delighted to share word of its special serenity and joys with readers of this book because even a lifetime later, this oasis of lovely flagstone paths and seasonal plantings remains unknown to many—including area residents. Tucked behind the Dyckman Farmhouse Museum, the garden is surrounded by the site's thick stone walls and towering foliage. As for the farmhouse and the family whose name it bears, the Dyckmans were loyal colony patriots, and when the British took over Manhattan, they fled, returning after the Revolutionary War ended. Uniforms of British troops and mercenary Hessians are on display, along with other artifacts of Colonial life. The white clapboard–and–stone house and little museum are quite charming, but for me, the real reason to visit is the garden.

↶ essentials
_____

⊟   4881 Broadway (at 204th Street), Manhattan 10034

✆   (212) 304-9422

🌐   dyckmanfarmhouse.org

$ Adults $1 (additional donations are appreciated); free for children under age 10

🕑   Wednesday–Saturday, 11 a.m.–4 p.m.; Sunday, noon–4 p.m.

🚌   **By subway:** A to 200th/Dyckman Street or 207th Street. **By bus:** M11 to 204th Street.

peaceful place 41

EAST POND, JAMAICA BAY WILDLIFE REFUGE
Jamaica Bay, Queens

CATEGORY ⌣ outdoor habitats ✪ ✪ ✪

*C*acti growing in the open in New York City? What a pleasant surprise. A few steps from the visitor center transport you to the Caribbean, with prickly pear cacti and thick ferns lining the sand and the packed dirt trail. I like to take the cutoff to Big John's Pond, a half-mile trek mostly on a boardwalk over a marshy wetland through bulrushes two stories high. The slightest breeze sets the bulrushes in motion, like a corps de ballet. At the end of the trail, there's a bird blind where you can take sneak peeks of colorful shorebirds, or just watch them preening or diving for snacks out in the open along the main trail. Even on a summer weekend, you are unlikely to pass more than a few other hikers, so it doesn't get much more peaceful than this, and it's all scented with salt air.

⌣ essentials

⌐≡⌐ Gateway National Recreation Area, Queens 11693

ⓒ (718) 318-4340

🌐 nps.gov/gate

$ Free admission

🕐 Visitors center: open daily, 8:30 a.m.–5 p.m. Trails: open daily, sunrise to sunset.

🚌 **By subway:** A to Broad Channel Station, then walk to Crossbay Boulevard and turn right (north) about a three-quarter mile to refuge.
By bus: Q21 or 53 to refuge.

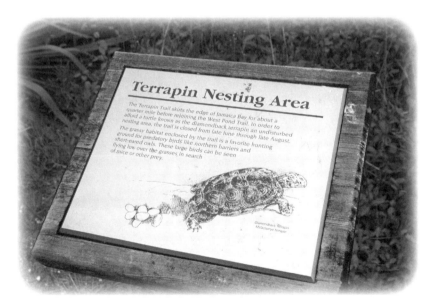

A large plaque describes the grassy habitat of the refuge

peaceful place 42

ELEVATED ACRE
Lower Manhattan

CATEGORY ⌣ urban surprises ✪ ✪

*I*t's easy to miss this sunny oasis because the entrance is virtually invisible. It's hidden in the shadow of a setback between two skyscrapers, and even if you do notice, it looks like a staircase and escalator to nowhere. So, consider this yet another secret spot revealed and shared. The escalator operates only on weekdays, so hardly anybody makes the three-flight climb on weekends, which is exactly when I enjoy visiting this little park. Mossy plantings and small shrubs are low enough not to interfere with the view overlooking the East River and several of its famous bridges, including the Brooklyn Bridge. Fortunately, the plantings also are dense enough to mask the drone of cars on the FDR Highway just below—although not the helicopters that seem to be landing and taking off an arm's reach away, at the Wall Street Heliport. If you descend the highway-side stairs and look back up at the building, you'll see some white streaks around the 15th floor that mark the spot of a longtime nest of a pair of peregrine falcons. In spring, bird-watchers hang out here, waiting for the chicks to take their first flight. Note that the space is available for rent for private parties and may not always be open to the public.

⌣ essentials

≡· 55 Water Street at Old Slip, Manhattan 10041

✆ (212) 747-9120   ◉ elevatedacre.com

$ Free admission   ◷ Open daily, 8 a.m.–8 p.m.

🚌 **By subway:** N or R to Whitehall Street; 2 or 3 to Wall Street.
By bus: M9 or 15 to Old Slip.

peaceful place 43

FLOYD BENNETT FIELD, GATEWAY NATIONAL RECREATION AREA

Flatbush, Brooklyn

CATEGORY ⌣ outdoor habitats ✪ ✪

*N*amed for the naval aviator who piloted Richard Byrd's historic flight over the North Pole in 1926, this airport played a significant role in early aviation history. It served such record-setting legends as Howard Hughes and Douglas "Wrong Way" Corrigan. These days, a part of the Gateway National Recreation Area, the hangars house historic aircraft, restoration projects, and an armed forces reserve center—and the runways are for bicycles instead of biplanes. But the North Forty Natural Area, between the runways and Mill Basin Inlet, is where you can lose yourself in the canopy of trees, dappled sunlight, and the sweet scent of honeysuckle. There are two grassy trails, shaped roughly like a figure eight. The lower Blue Trail loops past a pond with two bird blinds for sneak peeks of egrets and herons. The upper Red Trail is paved with bulrushes that hide all sense of city. Leashed dogs are permitted on the trails. In winter, the outer loop around both trails is popular with cross-country skiers.

⌣ essentials

▤ 50 Aviation Road, Brooklyn 11234

☎ (718) 338-3799   ⊕ nps.gov/gate $ Free admission

🕐 Hangar B: Tuesday, Thursday, and Saturday, 9 a.m.–4 p.m. National Park Service ranger station: Friday–Tuesday, 9 a.m.–5 p.m. Trails: open daily, sunrise to sunset.

🚌 **By subway:** A to Broad Channel Station, then walk to Crossbay Boulevard and turn right (north) about a three-quarter mile to refuge.
By bus: Q35 to Floyd Bennett Field–Aviator Sports Stop.

peaceful place 44

FOLEY SQUARE AND PAINE PARK
Lower Manhattan

CATEGORY ⌁ parks & gardens ✪ ✪

*O*ne side of this block-square park faces the grand facades of New York's two famous courthouses, with their broad steps and massive marble columns. In late morning, after the bustle of the start of the workday, both park and building steps are virtually empty, and you can sit on one of the benches and reflect on the inscription, "The true administration of justice is the firmest pillar of good government," carved into the pediment of the New York State Supreme Court. Or, you could ponder the wise sayings of Thomas Paine, the patriot whose writings in 1776 helped spark the American Revolution. My favorite quote of his is, "Lead, follow, or get out of the way." The park also features a tree-shaded portion with benches, and an open area dominated by a large fountain with several tiers suitable for perching, popular at lunchtime with brown-bagging office workers.

⌁ essentials

🖳	Duane to Worth streets, between Federal Plaza (Lafayette Street) and Foley Square (Centre Street); Manhattan 10007
✆	(212) 639-9675 🏵 nycgovparks.org/parks/M030
$	Free admission ⏱ Open daily, 5 a.m.–1 a.m.
🚌	**By subway:** J, M, or Z to City Hall; 6 to Brooklyn Bridge/City Hall. **By bus:** M22 to Foley Square.

peaceful place 45

FORBES GALLERIES

Greenwich Village, Lower Manhattan

CATEGORY ↝ museums & galleries ✪✪✪

Malcolm Forbes was a great collector. In fact, if he had not been so wealthy, he might have been called a pack rat. The magazine publisher amassed one of the world's largest armies of toy soldiers and extensive historic presidential memorabilia, among other things, and it's all on display here. Well, perhaps not all, as I'm sure there are goodies there's no room to showcase. This small museum inside the magazine's headquarters building is a sparkling jewel. Despite the worldwide fame of *Forbes* magazine, few people, including New Yorkers, seem to know the gallery exists. Thus the site is rarely crowded, except when the space is rented out for a charity fund-raiser. I find it soothing just to experience this eclectic collection of beautiful things that one man enjoyed and the family freely shares.

essentials

62 Fifth Avenue (at 12th Street), Manhattan 10011

(212) 206-5548 forbesgalleries.com

$ Free admission

Tuesday–Saturday, 10 a.m.–4 p.m. (Thursday by reservation only)

By subway: A, B, C, D, E, N, R, 1, 4, 5, or 6 to 14th Street.
By bus: M1, 2, 3, or 6 to 12th Street.

peaceful place 46

FORD FOUNDATION ATRIUM
Midtown Manhattan
CATEGORY ⌣ parks & gardens ✪ ✪ ✪

uilt in the 1960s for one of the largest philanthropic organizations in the
United States, this building quickly gained icon status for its open architecture and gardenlike terraced atrium. In some spots, the lush plantings resemble a jungle and totally block the sight of traffic passing on busy 42nd Street. I think of it as a small, urban greenhouse, with a tasteful babbling fountain that adds to the peacefulness. For the best view, climb the first few steps from the street, turn right (east), and perch on the ledge. Architects Kevin Roche and John Dinkeloo did not build in seating to invite lingering, so this space is usually empty.

⌣ essentials

≡	East 42nd Street between First and Second avenues, Manhattan 10017
✆	(212) 573-5000
🌐	fordfound.org
$	Free admission
🕙	Monday–Friday, 8 a.m.–4 p.m.
🚌	**By subway:** 4, 5, 6, or 7 to 42nd Street/Grand Central Station; walk east toward the United Nations. **By bus:** M104 or 42 to First Avenue; M15, 27, or 50 to 42nd Street.

peaceful place 47

FORT GREENE PARK

Fort Greene, Brooklyn

CATEGORY ⌣ parks & gardens ✪ ✪

esigned by Frederick Law Olmsted and Calvert Vaux in 1864, Fort Greene Park, known then as Washington Park, was Brooklyn's first major park, and is still one of its most lushly beautiful. That's in part because it is overshadowed by its larger neighbor, Prospect Park, also an Olmsted and Vaux design. There are pretty paths to wander, and harbor views from the top of the hill once afforded a splendid lookout in the Revolutionary War and the War of 1812. The poet Marianne Moore lived nearby, and my preferred place to perch is on a bench near the plaque in her honor, where I read her work—perhaps "Time, a substance / needful as an instance," from her poem "Black Earth." Another spot that invites introspection is the Prison Ship Martyrs Monument, which honors the 11,000 patriots from all 13 colonies who were imprisoned by the British aboard overcrowded ships in the harbor, and died of starvation and disease. Well, that is not a peaceful thought, but this is still a peaceful place.

⌣ essentials

Myrtle to DeKalb avenues, between Cumberland Street and Fort Greene Place; Brooklyn 11217

(212) 639-9675   nycgovparks.org/parks/fortgreenepark or fortgreenepark.org

$ Free admission   Open daily, 6 a.m.–1 a.m.

By subway: 2, 3, 4, 5, D, or N to Atlantic Avenue; C to Lafayette Avenue; G to Fulton Street; R, Q, or B to DeKalb Avenue. **By bus:** B38, 52, 25, or 26 to Fulton Street/Fort Greene Place.

peaceful place 48

FORT TILDEN, GATEWAY NATIONAL RECREATION AREA

Breezy Point, Queens

CATEGORY ↙ outdoor habitats ✪ ✪

*K*eep walking west past the end of the boardwalk and the park border at Jacob Riis Park to this former military base on the tip of the Rockaway Peninsula, where you can still find the concrete bases for battleship guns that guarded New York Harbor through two world wars. It's a one-mile amble from the Riis Park bathhouse to the observation deck here, the highest point on the peninsula. After the boardwalk ends, stay along the beach until you get to an unmarked sandy trail inland. Follow it past a small freshwater pond to a set of wooden stairs to the overlook, where, truly, on a clear day you can see forever into the Atlantic in one direction and to the Lower Manhattan skyline in the distance in another. There's also a paved road within Fort Tilden. The road is closed to cars from mid-June to mid-September and is popular with bicyclists.

↙ essentials

⊟ Atlantic Ocean on the tip of Rockaway Peninsula, Queens 11697

✆ (718) 318-4300   ◉ nyharborparks.org/visit/foti.html or nps.gov/gate

$ Free admission

◔ Open daily, sunrise to sunset

🚌 **By subway and bus:** 2 or 5 to Flatbush Avenue, then the Q35 bus to the Jacob Riis Park entrance; or the A train to Rockaway Park, then bus Q25 or Q22 to the park entrance. New York Water Taxi (212-742-1969) offers weekend service from Wall Street, Pier 11, and Brooklyn Army Terminal to Riis Landing in season.

peaceful place 49

FORT TOTTEN PARK
Bay Terrace, Queens

CATEGORY ⌣ outdoor habitats ✪ ✪

*V*ictorian lampposts and stately Victorian wood-sided and brick buildings with wrap-around columned porches? These embellishments will make you think you have been transported to Savannah, Georgia, or Charleston, South Carolina—except for the northern oaks and maples standing in for the southern live oaks. The original fort consists of the 10-acre park, as well as surrounding facilities now being used by the Fire Department of New York City, NYPD, EMS, and the Bayside Historical Society. Otherwise, this destination offers canoeing, bird-watching, and broad, traffic-free streets for bicycling, jogging, or long walks with or without Fido—leashed only.

My preferred spot is past the old parade grounds and the gazebo. I like to sit on a bench on Shore Road, overlooking the Little Neck Bay inlet of Long Island Sound, and listen to gently lapping water. I always stop by the visitor center for a journey into the past, as Fort Totten was built to defend New York Harbor in the 1860s. The center was an ordinance house storing weaponry during the Civil War. Now it showcases small displays of uniforms, photos, and replica artillery. Behind the building, tucked into the hillside, are the amazing arched caverns of King Battery, which once held live arms. Other than an occasional ice-cream truck at the park entrance, there's no food or water here, so be sure to bring your own. In fact, I suggest a good picnic, which you, too, can enjoy overlooking the sound.

⌣ essentials

✉ Cross Island Parkway, between Totten Avenue and 15th Road; Queens 11359

✆ (718) 352-1769

nycgovparks.org/parks/forttotten

$ Free admission

Open daily, 5 a.m.–1 a.m.

By subway and bus: 7 to Flushing/Main Street (last stop), then the Q13 or 16 bus to park entrance (last stop).

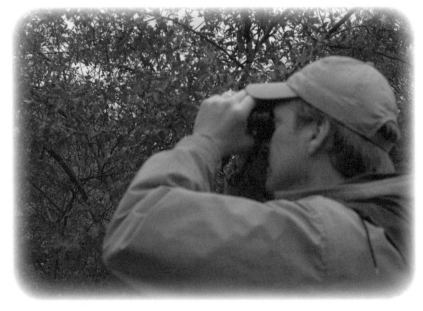

Many city parks offer areas for bird-watching.

peaceful place 50

FORT TRYON PARK
Washington Heights, Northern Manhattan
CATEGORY ⌣ parks & gardens ✪ ✪

ike the Cloisters, which is located within Fort Tryon, the parkland was a gift to the city from the Rockefeller family. And what a gift—66 hilltop acres! Frederick Law Olmsted Jr., son of the co-architect of Central Park and Brooklyn's Prospect Park, landscaped the setting with endless elms and low-growing heather. Take your pick of any of the shaded walking paths that wind up to the Cloisters from Broadway, or downhill from the flagpole at Linden Terrace. Atop the park, stroll the broad promenade alongside and high above the Hudson River. Walk south, and tune into the rhythmic hum of traffic crossing the George Washington Bridge just ahead. Be sure to stop by the New Leaf Restaurant and Bar, housed in a 1930s cottage—One Margaret Corbin Drive, (212) 568-5323, www.nyrp.org/newleaf. A five-minute walk south from the Cloisters (see page 51), the cafe offers its patio garden from April to October. Entertainer Bette Midler operates it through her New York Restoration Project, a nonprofit group that beautifies New York City parks and gardens.

⌣ essentials

▭   Broadway to Riverside Drive, between West 192nd and Dyckman streets; Manhattan 10040

✆   (212) 795-1388   🐦 nycgovparks.org/parks/forttryonpark

$ Free admission   🕙 Open daily, 5 a.m.–1 a.m.

🚌   **By subway:** A to 190th Street or Dyckman Street.
By bus: M4 to the Cloisters, in Fort Tryon Park; M98 to 193rd Street.

peaceful place 51

GOVERNORS ISLAND
Lower Manhattan

CATEGORY ◡ historic sites ✪

For more than 200 years, from 1776 to 1996, this island off the southern tip of Manhattan served as a fortress protecting New York Harbor from invaders. In the 1960s, the island became the largest U.S. Coast Guard base in the world. It's also been a world summit site: This is where President Reagan hosted U.S.S.R. president Mikhail Gorbachev in 1988. I wonder if the two leaders took a break and walked to the grassy lawn on the south side of the island, now called Picnic Point, for a close-up view of the Statue of Liberty best described as "in your face." It's the absolute highlight of the 2.2-mile waterfront road that now rings the island, and is therefore popular with weekend walkers and cyclists.

So, if you want solitude, head to the island's western side. That view across Buttermilk Channel to the Brooklyn Bridge will transfix you, as will the gossamer cables shimmering in the sunshine. Avoid summer evenings when there's a rock concert on the sandy Water Taxi Beach. Lucky for us, the feds sold the island in 2003 to New York City for $1 to turn it into public parkland. That was an even better deal than a Dutch businessman negotiated when he bought the island from the local Manahattas tribe in 1637 for two ax heads, beads, and nails. And we are lucky, too, that the seven-minute ferry ride is free. If you don't have your own bicycle, you can rent one on the island, but if you want to go fishing, you have to bring your own gear, and it's catch-and-release only.

⌣ essentials

⌐≡⌐   Governors Island Ferry: Battery Maritime Building, 10 South Street, Manhattan 10005

☏   (212) 825-3045

🌐   govisland.com or nps.gov/gois

$ Free admission

🕐   Late May to mid-October: Friday, 10 a.m.–5 p.m.; Saturday–Sunday, 10 a.m.–7 p.m.; later on concert evenings

🚌   **By subway:** 1 to South Ferry; 4 or 5 to Bowling Green; R or W to Whitehall Street. **By bus:** M1, 6, 9, or 15. The Governors Island Ferry departs from the Battery Maritime Building next to the Staten Island Ferry Terminal. Ferries leave at least once an hour on Friday, 10 a.m.–3 p.m. and Saturday–Sunday, 10 a.m.–5 p.m.

peaceful place 52

GRAND FERRY PARK
Williamsburg, Brooklyn
CATEGORY ↵ scenic vistas ✪

For most of the 1800s, this was a hectic spot as the Brooklyn terminal for ferries departing every five minutes for the Lower East Side of Manhattan. They were replaced by the Williamsburg Bridge and the subway in the early 1900s. Now, this lovely little oasis of shady river birch and locust trees, flower plantings, and brick walkways is used mostly by car service drivers hanging out between fares and workers from the adjoining warehouses on lunchtime breaks. Pity, because this waterfront park has glorious views of Manhattan across the East River, especially at sunset. Just don't linger much longer. It's well worth the ten-minute walk from the nearest subway, and you'll pass one of the world's legendary steakhouses, where you can fortify yourself with something thick and, preferably, medium-rare. Peter Luger has been satisfying carnivores since 1887—178 Broadway, (718) 387-7400, peterluger.com, open daily for lunch and dinner.

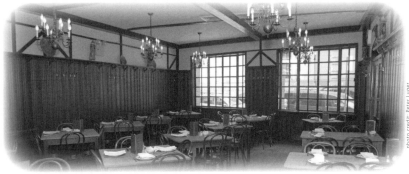

Dining room at Peter Luger

⌄ essentials

- 📧   Grand Street to West River Street on the East River, Brooklyn 11211

- 📞   (212) 639-9675

- 🌐   nycgovparks.org/parks/B401

- $ Free admission

- 🕐   Open daily, 6 a.m.–1 a.m., but not recommended after sunset

- 🚌   **By subway:** J, M, or Z to Marcy Avenue; G to Broadway.
  By bus: Q59 to Grand Street.

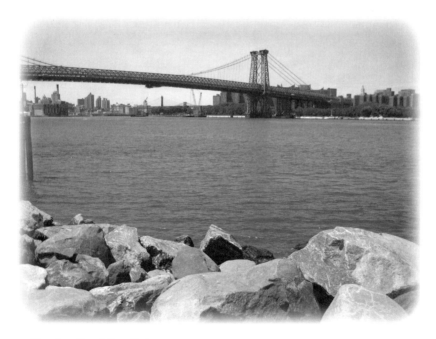

View from Grand Ferry Park

peaceful place 53

GREENACRE PARK
Midtown Manhattan

CATEGORY ↙ urban surprises ✪

*A*nother tiny slice of green tucked between midtown skyscrapers, this vest-pocket park features a two-story waterfall that masks street noises and offers a cooling spray on hot summer days when the wind is right. Another calming feature is the small brook that runs along the east wall. There are plenty of tables and chairs that can be moved about to make the most of the ever-changing path of sunlight through neighboring buildings. Of course, this open-air escape is crowded at lunchtime on warm-weather days with brown-bagging office workers, so go any other time.

↙ essentials

📧 217 East 51st Street (between Second and Third avenues), Manhattan 10022

📞 (212) 838-0528 or (212) 649-5691

🌐 No Web site

$ Free admission

🕐 Open daily, sunrise to sunset

🚇 **By subway:** 6 to 51st Street; E or F to 53rd Street.
    By bus: M27 or 50 to Second or Third Avenue; M101, 102, or 103 to 51st Street.

peaceful place 54

GREENBELT NATURE CENTER, S. I. GREENBELT
Sea View, Staten Island

CATEGORY ⌣ outdoor habitats ✪ ✪

hirty-five miles of hiking and multiuse bike trails thread through these 2,800 acres of forests, meadows, ponds, hills, and valleys, all in the middle of Staten Island. So you are more likely to see birds and butterflies than to run into other people. Even though trails are well marked and well maintained for the most part, there are some rocky, slippery, and otherwise treacherous portions that you just might not expect in the middle of a New York City borough. My advice: good hiking boots.

The Greenbelt Nature Center staff offers trail maps and friendly advice. They likely will tell you to start on the Blue Trail behind the building, to hook up with the easy, four-mile loop of the Red Trail. That trail passes close to Heyerdahl Hill, named for the owner of a house that used to be here; the stone steps, which you will see, are all that remain. The Red Trail is a loop trail; on most others, you will be hiking out-and-backs that travel east to west or north to south. From the Red Trail, you can take the cutoff to Historic Richmond Town, a living-history village and museum where you'll wind up in the 17th and 18th centuries. That isn't a bad thing, except when the place is noisy with schoolchildren. Avoid any Tuesday when school is in session, which is school day at the Nature Center.

⌣ essentials

⌸ 700 Rockland Avenue (at Brielle Avenue), Staten Island 10314

☏ (718) 351-3450   ✈ sigreenbelt.org $ Free admission

☉ Nature Center: April–October: Tuesday–Sunday, 10 a.m.–5 p.m. November–March: Wednesday–Sunday, 11 a.m.–5 p.m. Trails: open daily, sunrise to sunset.

🚌 **By bus:** From the Staten Island Ferry Terminal, take S74 to Rockland Avenue; transfer to the S54 or 57 to Brielle Avenue.

peaceful place 55

GREEN-WOOD CEMETERY
Bay Ridge, Brooklyn

CATEGORY ◡ spiritual enclaves ❂ ❂

ive ponds alive with mallards and geese, rolling hills dotted with some of the most mature trees in Brooklyn favored by all manner of songbirds, and serpentine walkways without cars or bicycles make up this park/cemetery. Designed in 1838, Green-Wood is half the size of Central Park, but just as full of wonder. It is on the National Register of Historic Places, and it also happens to contain some 500,000 souls. They include such world-famous occupants as artist Louis Comfort Tiffany, inventor Samuel Morse, and artists Currier and Ives—Nathaniel and James Merritt, respectively. My odyssey leads me to the grave of Charles Ebbetts, owner of the beloved Brooklyn Dodgers. Ebbets Field was a few blocks from where an aunt and uncle of mine lived, and pausing with the memory of Mr. Ebbetts lets me reflect on my childhood Sunday visits to them. I would sit at an open living room window listening to the roars of the baseball crowd. I also like to pay respects to Leonard Bernstein and Henry E. Steinway Jr. to muse on the pleasure of their music.

◡ essentials

✉	500 25th Street (at Fifth Avenue), Brooklyn 11232
☏	(718) 768-7300 ⊕ green-wood.com
$	Free admission for self-guided tours (get a map at the entrance); guided trolley tours (every Wednesday at 1 p.m.) $15; guided walking tours $10
⊙	Open daily, 8 a.m.–5 p.m.
🚃	**By subway:** R to 25th Street, then walk one block to the entrance.

peaceful place 56

HALL OF FAME FOR GREAT AMERICANS COLONNADE

University Heights, Bronx

CATEGORY ↩ historic sites ✪ ✪ ✪

When I was a kid, this was the Bronx campus of New York University, which built the grand colonnade in 1901 to honor great Americans and inspire students. Now Bronx Community College, the campus still teems with college life as part of the city's famed university system, and the original, grand Beaux Arts buildings still impress. Then as now, the students generally ignore the colonnade, despite its inspiring collection of about 100 bronze busts, with beautiful architectural details. The lineup is thought-provoking, as your mind jumps from one historic period and accomplishment to another: Franklin Delano Roosevelt is near John Philip Sousa; Thomas Edison is close

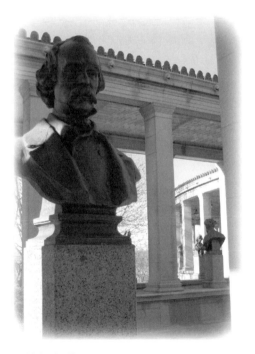

Nathaniel Hawthorne, one of almost 100 bronze busts of famous historic figures

to brothers Wilbur and Orville Wright; another section holds inventors Samuel Morse, Alexander Graham Bell, and Eli Whitney. My favorites, though, are Henry David Thoreau, whose book about life in the woods at Walden Pond speaks volumes about serenity, and Walt Whitman, whose poetry about leaves and grass still thrills. Another bonus for making your way here: Between the stately columns, the colonnade offers dramatic views of Manhattan from one of the highest points in the Bronx.

⌣ essentials

✉	2155 University Avenue, Bronx 10453
✆	(718) 289-5161
🌐	bcc.cuny.edu/halloffame
$	Free admission
🕐	Open daily, 9 a.m.–5 p.m.
🚇	**By subway:** 4 to Burnside Avenue. **By bus:** Bx3, Bx40, or Bx42.

peaceful place 57

HARLEM MEER, CENTRAL PARK
Upper Manhattan

CATEGORY ⌣ parks & gardens ✪ ✪ ✪

A leisurely stroll around this amoeba-shaped meer (Dutch for "lake") can restore you in about a half-hour. But stay longer to appreciate the sight and sound of migrating birds and the thickets of seasonal flowers around some of the oldest oak, beech, and bald-cypress trees in Central Park. Take your seat on any of the benches scattered around the perimeter, but for the prime vista, choose a bench that faces into the park, just inside the Fifth Avenue stone wall. From here, you'll look across sparkling Harlem Meer to the rock outcroppings on its western edge. Very peaceful, indeed. If your thoughts meander to some exercise, cast your eyes to the lakeshore's Charles A. Dana Discovery Center. The handsome Victorian-style building serves as the starting point for free guided walking tours.

⌣ essentials

🖃 Fifth Avenue from 106th to 110th Street, Manhattan 10026

✆ (212) 310-6600; Charles A. Dana Discovery Center: (212) 860-1370

🌐 centralparknyc.org $ Free admission

🕐 Open daily, 6 a.m.–1 a.m., but not recommended after sunset. Charles A. Dana Discovery Center: April–October: Tuesday–Sunday, 10 a.m.–5 p.m. November–March: Wednesday–Sunday, 10 a.m.–5 p.m.

🚌 **By subway:** 2, 3, or 6 to 110th Street; B or C to Cathedral Parkway/110th Street. **By bus:** M1, 2, 3, 4, or 96 to 105th Street.

peaceful place 58

HEIGHTS BOOKS
Brooklyn Heights, Brooklyn

CATEGORY ↵ shops & services ⊕ ⊕

*F*rom $1 bargains to rare first editions or signed art books for collectors
—with science fiction, mystery, biography, and philosophy books in between—
this fiercely independent used-book store is a neighborhood staple with a loyal customer
following. The youthful owner prides herself on hiring only overqualified staff, such as an
adjunct professor at New York Law School who has written or edited 20 books himself.
The shelves are crowded with hard covers and paperbacks side by side, and the store is
just a bit cramped, but it's still a private and contemplative space—well deserving of two
stars for peacefulness.

↵ essentials

≡ 120 Smith Street, Brooklyn 11201

☏ (718) 624-4876

⊕ heightsbooks.com

$ Free admission

☼ Monday–Thursday, 11 a.m.–9 p.m.; Friday–Saturday, 11 a.m.–10 p.m.;
Sunday, noon–9 p.m.

🚇 **By subway:** 2 or 3, M or R to Court Street; A, C, or F to Jay Street/Borough Hall.

peaceful place 59

HIGH LINE
West Side, Lower Manhattan

CATEGORY ⌣ scenic vistas ✪ ✪

The last train ran on an elevated rail line here in 1980, and it took nearly 30 years for local activists to succeed in turning this abandoned eyesore into a lovely elevated park. In 2009, the first section of this strip of green 30 feet above the ground opened. It extends from Gansevoort Street in the Meatpacking District to 20th Street, between 10th and 11th avenues. When completed, it will be open all the way to 34th Street. Already, nearly every step has drop-dead views of the Hudson River and the Midtown and Lower Manhattan skylines. The cityscape is interspersed with lush plantings and a water feature to muffle the sound of the West Side Highway just below. There are plenty of seats and viewing platforms to use for relaxing and enjoying the river views. They are infinitely more tranquil than the cacophony of ego-architecture, some actually straddling the High Line, casting nasty shadows and screaming, "Look at me." For serenity, look away. Even so, the High Line is a bicycle-free alternative to Hudson River Park a few steps away. My favorite time to visit—for the solitude, the breeze, and the sunset—is a crisp spring or fall afternoon. Another good time: a summer morning, before late-sleeping locals arrive.

⌣ essentials

✉ Access the High Line along 10th Avenue at Gansevoort, 14th, 16th, 18th, or 20th streets; Manhattan 10011

☎ (212) 500-6035   🌐 thehighline.org $ Free admission

🕐 Open daily, 7 a.m.–10 p.m. in summer; 7 a.m.–8 p.m. in winter

🚌 **By subway:** 1, 2, 3, L, C, E, or A to 14th Street, then walk to the park just past 10th Avenue; 1 to 23rd Street. **By bus:** M11 to Washington Street or Ninth Avenue; M14 to Ninth Avenue; M23 or 34 to 10th Avenue.

peaceful place 60

HUDSON RIVER PARK

West Side, Midtown and Lower Manhattan

CATEGORY ⌣ parks & gardens ✪ ✪ ✪

*E*ven after 20 years, this is still a work in progress. The goal is to connect pieces of riverside parkland from the Battery to 59th Street, refurbish abandoned piers, and create a continuous, smooth, multiuse asphalt route for walking, bicycling, and inline skating. The section between Houston and Charles streets is the most lush, with flower plantings and trees shading walking paths, and it is relatively unoccupied on weekdays. But even on busy, warm-weather weekends, there's still a spot of solitude on the lawn on the south side of Pier 40, where you can watch kayakers. This is one of three Hudson River piers where Downtown Boathouse (downtownboathouse. org) offers free kayaking on weekends, mid-May to mid-October. It's a gloriously serene experience to dip a paddle into the water, propel yourself silently, and be further calmed by the views from this watery perspective.

⌣ essentials

☐ Battery Street to 59th Street, at the Hudson River; Manhattan 10019, 10018, 10001, 10011, 10014, 10013, 10007, 10280

☎ (212) 627-2020   🌐 hudsonriverpark.org

$ Free admission   🕐 Open daily, 6 a.m.–1 a.m.

🚌 **By subway:** 1, 2, or 3 between South Ferry and 59th Street, and then the appropriate cross-town bus to river.

peaceful place 61

IDLEWILD BOOKS
Chelsea, Lower Manhattan

CATEGORY ⌣ shops & services ✪ ✪ ✪

*S*unlight spilling through the massive windows of a second-story loftlike space turns this eclectic bookshop into a soul-enriching escape. Idlewild Books specializes in travel guidebooks, so you can explore the world by browsing the shelves. Moreover, many country sections have biographies of famous native sons and daughters, or literary works by writers from those countries. So the Russia section could include a bio on Vladimir Putin, while the Argentina section holds titles by world-renowned Jorge Luis Borges. A scattering of sofas and chairs invites getting cozy with a good country. There's also a selection of tabletop globes to spin, and a friendly, well-traveled young staff for a bit of chatting if you are in the mood.

⌣ essentials

⌨ 12 West 19th Street, Manhattan 10011

✆ (212) 414-8888

🌐 idlewildbooks.com

$ Free admission

🕐 Monday–Friday, 11:30 a.m.–8 p.m.; Saturday–Sunday, noon–7 p.m.

🚌 **By subway:** 1 to 18th Street; D to 23rd Street.
By bus: M14 or 23 to Fifth Avenue.

peaceful place 62

INWOOD HILL PARK
Northern Manhattan

CATEGORY ↙ parks & gardens ✪ ✪ ✪

N obody really knows exactly where Peter Minuit purchased the entire island from the local Lenape tribe for $24 worth of trinkets, but a plaque says it was here, on this rocky, hilly northern tip of Manhattan. Here also, the Harlem River flows into the Hudson, and the currents and whirlpools prompted the Colonial Dutch settlers to name it Spuyten Duyvil, or spitting devil. But the residential area surrounding Inwood Hill remains bucolic, and shaded walking paths lace the park's natural forest—the last one on the island. To really unwind, head north and west from the park's ball fields until you reach a V-shaped walkway lined with benches. There, you can contemplate a soothing panorama: the towering cliffs of the Palisades across the Hudson River, the thickly forested northern edge of Fort Tryon Park, and seagulls and mallards pecking and preening by Manhattan's only salt-marsh pond. The immense and graceful arch of the Henry Hudson Bridge spans across Spuyten Duyvil Creek. The modern apartments of the Riverdale section of the Bronx rise to your right. And you'll hear the silvery Metro-North commuter train speeding along the Bronx's waterfront.

When you are ready to reconnect, walk over to the welcoming Inwood Hill Nature Center housed in a turquoise-and-white tiled building built by the WPA. Then stop in for a homemade pastry or soup at Indian Road Café & Market—600 West 218th Street, (212) 942-7451, indianroadcafe.com. It's the kind of friendly, slightly Bohemian neighborhood place you would hope to find in the Montparnasse section of Paris or in San Francisco's Haight-Ashbury neighborhood.

essentials

Seaman Avenue to Hudson River, between West 207th Street to West 218th Street and Harlem River; Manhattan 10034

(212) 304-2365   nycgovparks.org/parks/inwoodhillpark

$ Free admission

Open daily, 6 a.m.–1 a.m. Nature center: Wednesday–Sunday, 11 a.m.–4 p.m.

By subway: A to 207th Street (last stop); 1 to 215th Street.
By bus: M100, Bx7, Bx12, or Bx20 to 207th Street.

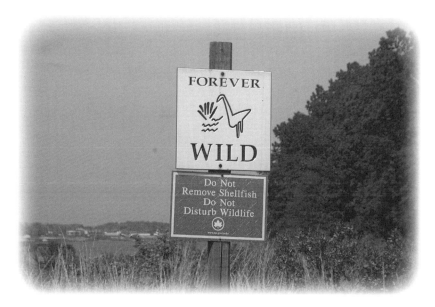

Signage at Manhattan's only salt-marsh pond

peaceful place 63

IRIS AND B. GERALD CANTOR ROOF GARDEN, METROPOLITAN MUSEUM OF ART

Upper Manhattan

CATEGORY ⌣ scenic vistas ✪

B. Gerald Cantor and his wife, Iris, avidly collected fine art, especially Auguste Rodin sculptures. An impressive collection, the sculptures range in size from tabletop to the equivalent of a small car, and some even dot this ethereal space on the fifth floor of the Metropolitan Museum of Art. Mr. Cantor co-founded the global securities firm Cantor Fitzgerald, and those offices in the World Trade Center were demolished on September 11, 2001—costing the lives of hundreds of the company's employees and destroying priceless art.

Once you have oohed and ahhed over the garden's sculptures, which change depending on the exhibits, you can move on to the sweeping views across Central Park and Midtown. The setting is magical just before sunset, but enough people know about that; so the best time to visit and have it all to yourself is in the morning, shortly after the museum opens. May through autumn, every day except Mondays, the roof garden cafe starts serving at 10, so you can pair a light snack and steaming cup of coffee or tea with your view.

⌣ essentials

▤	1000 Fifth Avenue (at 82nd Street), Manhattan 10028
☎	(212) 535-7710 🌐 metmuseum.org
$	Suggested contribution (includes access to all museum buildings and exhibits): adults $20; seniors $15; students $10; free for members, children under age 12, and New York City public school students
🕐	Open Sunday and Tuesday–Thursday, 10 a.m.–4:30 p.m.; Friday–Saturday, 10 a.m.–8:30 p.m.
🚌	**By subway:** 4, 5, or 6 to 86th Street; walk three blocks west to Fifth Avenue. **By bus:** M1, 2, 3, or 4 to 82nd Street; M86 to Fifth Avenue.

peaceful place 64

ISAMU NOGUCHI GARDEN MUSEUM
Long Island City, Queens
CATEGORY 〜 parks & gardens ✪ ✪ ✪

A nondescript building in a waterfront warehouse area shelters one of the most tranquil spots in the city. Contemplation accompanies each step around any of the 200-plus sculptures by the famed artist and interior designer Isamu Noguchi. Marble, metal, wood, and clay creations large and small fan out in this massive space. Benches are scattered throughout the galleries and garden, so you can linger and admire

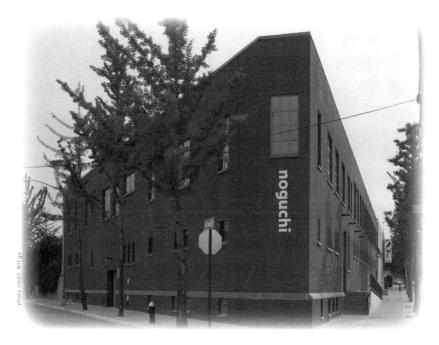

photo credit: NYCgo

Exterior of sculpture-filled Isamu Noguchi Garden Museum

Noguchi's chiseled shapes and his use of the natural patterns in stone and wood. For me, the outdoor garden space is even more peaceful, especially when puffy clouds dot the sky and throw patterns of light and shadow. The only crowded time is early afternoon, for the free 2 p.m. docent tour.

essentials

9-01 33rd Road (at Vernon Boulevard), Queens 11106

(718) 204-7088

noguchi.org

Adults $10; seniors and students $5; free for members, children under age 12, and New York City public school students

Wednesday–Friday, 10 a.m.–5 p.m.; Saturday–Sunday, 11 a.m.–6 p.m.

By subway: N or W to Broadway (in Queens), then walk ten blocks toward the Manhattan skyline and East River to Vernon Boulevard and turn left to the museum. Or F to Queensbridge/21st Street, then take the Q69 bus to Broadway and walk about five minutes toward the Manhattan skyline and East River to Vernon Boulevard, then left to the museum. Wednesday–Friday, take 7 to Vernon-Jackson in Queens, walk one block north on Vernon toward 50th Avenue, and take the Q103 bus in front of the Brasil Coffee House to 33rd Road. After exiting, turn right and make an immediate left onto 33rd Road. On Sundays, there is a shuttle bus from the Asia Society, at Park Avenue and 70th Street in Manhattan ($5 each way) from 12:30 p.m.–3:30 p.m. each hour.

peaceful place 65

JACOB RIIS PARK, GATEWAY NATIONAL RECREATION AREA

Rockaway, Queens

CATEGORY ↵ outdoor habitats ✪ ✪ ✪

A great, turreted Art Deco bathhouse built in the Works Progress Administration days of the 1930s once stood guard over lovers of sun, sand, surf, and solitude. These days, it houses the visitor center of the National Park Service, where you can find maps, friendly advice, and displays of historical photos from the 1930s to the 1960s, but no showers or lockers. When I was a kid, we stayed at beach sections close to the boardwalk ice cream concessions. Now, I prefer the more isolated areas on the west (right) side of the bathhouse. Sections from Number 10 to the park border at Number 17 have wild dunes and nobody nearby to kick sand on your reverie, but there's also no swimming here because there are no lifeguards beyond Number 9. I also enjoy the dedicated section for kite flying because the colorful, fluttering shapes in the sky and the happy shouts of children attached to incredibly long strings make me smile.

↵ essentials

⊟   Rockaway Beach Boulevard, Queens 11697

✆   (718) 318-4300   ⦿ nyharborparks.org/visit/jari.html or nps.gov/gate

$ Free admission   🕐 Open daily, 9 a.m.–5 p.m.

🚌   **By subway:** 2 or 5 to Flatbush Avenue, then the Q35 bus to park entrance; or the A or S to Rockaway Park, then the Q35 or Q22 bus to the park entrance. New York Water Taxi [(212) 742-1969, rockawayferry.com, $6 one-way) offers weekday commuter and summer weekend service from Wall Street, Pier 11, and the Brooklyn Army Terminal to Riis Landing.

peaceful place 66

JACQUES MARCHAIS MUSEUM OF TIBETAN ART
Lighthouse Hill, Staten Island
CATEGORY ↩ museums & galleries ✪ ✪ ✪

*I*t's easy to miss the unmarked wooden gate to this little treasure, on a street populated by several homes that could pass for Tony Soprano's luxurious spread. Those properties, however, arrived decades after 1945, when a female art dealer and collector of Asian works named Jacques Marchais built this remarkable rough stone hideaway into the side of a hill. Built to resemble a Tibetan temple, the site's pieces include a rare sand mandala by a monk from Bhutan, plus Buddha statues in various sizes from Tibet, Nepal, and Mongolia, some from the 16th century. Silk brocade throw pillows on the benches inside invite reflection, as does the outdoor meditation garden, which is dotted with colorful Tibetan prayer flags and dwarf pines in odd shapes that invite yet more thought. I like sitting on one of the stone benches, enchanted by the wind chimes and the dappled sunlight through the trees. Even winter has a special appeal, when a dusting of snow makes this magical place seem surreal. Yes, the Dalai Lama has visited; no, he did not participate in the yoga classes and meditation workshops held here.

↩ essentials

✉   338 Lighthouse Avenue, Staten Island 10306

☎   (718) 987-3500

🌐   tibetanmuseum.org

$ Adults $5; seniors and students $3; free for members and children under age 6

April–November: Wednesday–Sunday, 1 p.m.–5 p.m. (Sunday's last admission at 4:30 p.m.)
December–March: Thursday–Sunday, 1 p.m.–5 p.m. (Sunday's last admission at 4:30 p.m.)

By bus: Staten Island Ferry to St. George Terminal, then S74 to Lighthouse Avenue; walk up the hill (5–10 minutes) to the museum. S79 at Fourth Avenue and 86th Street in Brooklyn to Clove Road/Targee Street; walk one block to Richmond Road, then transfer to S74. Debark at Lighthouse Avenue, and walk up the hill to the museum.

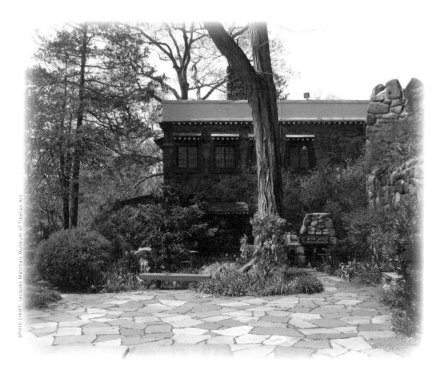

photo credit: Jacques Marchais Museum of Tibetan Art

Garden at Jacques Marchais Museum of Tibetan Art

peaceful place 67

JAPANESE HILL-AND-POND GARDEN, BROOKLYN BOTANIC GARDEN

Park Slope, Brooklyn

CATEGORY ⌣ parks & gardens ✪ ✪ ✪

*A*void the covered overlook area immediately in front of the entrance, which tends to get crowded, to walk around the pond. Each step is a new vista of stone lanterns; shrubs pruned into pleasing shapes; turtles, some as large as dinner plates, sunning themselves on the rocks; and brightly colored koi, some as large as Pacific salmon. Always, the famous red and black Torii arch is in view, sometimes decorated with a cormorant or two. There are few benches here, but the low log fence bordering the pond side path provides excellent seating for contemplation. The least crowded time to visit this most popular part of the park is weekday mornings.

⌣ essentials

✉	900 Washington Avenue, Brooklyn 11225 (Entrances are on Eastern Parkway adjoining the Brooklyn Museum; Flatbush Avenue at Empire Boulevard; and Washington Avenue.)
☎	(718) 623-7200 🌐 bbg.org
$	Adults $8; seniors and students $4; free for members and children under age 12; free for seniors on Fridays; free on Tuesdays, Saturdays until noon, and Monday–Friday mid-November to February
🕐	Mid-March to October: Tuesday–Friday, 8 a.m.–6 p.m.; Saturday–Sunday and some holiday Mondays, 10 a.m.–6 p.m. November to mid-March: Tuesday–Friday, 8 a.m.–4:30 p.m.; Saturday–Sunday and some holiday Mondays, 10 a.m.–4:30 p.m.
🚌	**By subway:** 2 or 3 to Eastern Parkway; B, Q, or S to Prospect Park. **By bus:** B71 to the museum; B48 to Franklin Avenue and Eastern Parkway.

peaceful place 68

JEFFERSON MARKET BRANCH LIBRARY
Greenwich Village, Lower Manhattan

CATEGORY ↵ reading rooms ✪ ✪ ✪

he Jeff, as local residents call the library, is not just quiet, but also gorgeous. This Victorian Gothic gem was voted one of the ten most beautiful buildings in America in the 1880s. It was built as a courthouse in the 1870s, and one of the architects was Calvert Vaux, more famous for the role he played in the design of Central Park. The Jeff's wide, winding stone staircase, lit by enormous stained-glass windows, leads to a grand reading room with a ceiling that is almost 40 feet high. Here, too, are carved wood doorways, and yet more soaring stained-glass windows that let in plenty of light, even when skies are gray. This is a wonderful, restful place to unwind, with or without your laptop. There's free Wi-Fi and a table with plenty of outlets. Actually, forget the laptop and escape into the past with one of this branch library's extensive collection of New York City history books, including tomes about famous local trials.

Historical tidbit: One case tried here concerned the murder of architect Stanford White, who built another famous New York landmark—the Washington Arch, a few blocks away. Harry Kendall Thaw, the jealous husband of White's ex-paramour, show-girl Evelyn Nesbit, took the architect's life and was found not guilty by reason of insanity in the most famous scandal and trial of its time. But that is decidedly unpeaceful, so perhaps it's best not to stray into such reports while you are seeking tranquility here.

↵ essentials

▭ 425 Sixth Avenue (Avenue of the Americas at 10th Street), Manhattan 10011

 (212) 243-4334

nypl.org/branch/local/man/jmr.cfm

$ Free admission

Open Monday and Wednesday, 9 a.m.–8 p.m.; Tuesday and Thursday, 9 a.m.–7 p.m.; Friday–Saturday, 10 a.m.–5 p.m.

By subway: F, A, C, or E to Fourth Street (use Waverly Place exit); 2 or 3 to 12th Street; 1 to Christopher Street. **By bus:** M2, 3, or 5 to Tenth Street; M8 to Eighth Street.

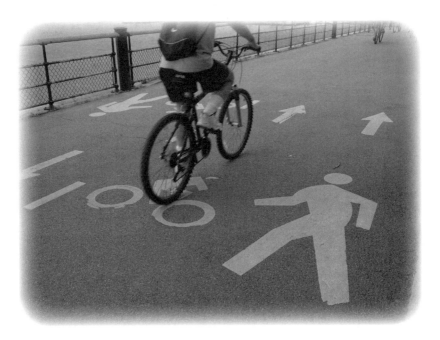

Enjoy New York City by foot or bicycle.

peaceful place 69

JOHN FINLEY WALK, CARL SCHURZ PARK
Upper East Side, Upper Manhattan

CATEGORY ↶ scenic vistas ✪ ✪ ✪

I f the soaring symmetry of bridges calms and restores you, then take your place at the top of the stone staircase at the eastern end of 86th Street, which takes you to a promenade built atop FDR Drive. The view includes the Robert F. Kennedy Memorial/ Triborough Bridge, the Queensboro/59th Street Bridge, and Amtrak's Hell Gate Bridge. It's a calm refuge any hour of day, but my favorite time is before local residents come home from work and walk their dogs here. While Mayor Michael Bloomberg lives in a town house nearby, the official mayoral residence, Gracie Mansion, is at the northern end of the park. Used primarily for fundraisers, city events, and tours, the mansion's hosting of various activities does not abridge the peacefulness of the John Finley Walk.

↶ essentials

🖃 East End Avenue to East River, between East 84th and East 90th streets, Manhattan 10128

☎ Park: (212) 459-4455; Gracie Mansion: (212) 639-9675

🌐 nycgovparks.org/parks/carlschurz or carlschurzparknyc.org

$ Free admission. Gracie Mansion: adults $7, seniors $4; free for students

🕐 Open daily, 6 a.m.–1 a.m. (Reservations required for mansion tours.)

🚌 **By subway:** 4, 5, or 6 to 86th Street.
    By bus: M79 to East End Avenue; M86 to York Avenue; M15 or M31 to 86th Street.

peaceful place 70

JOHN MUIR NATURE TRAIL, VAN CORTLANDT PARK
Riverdale and North Bronx, Bronx

CATEGORY ⌣ outdoor habitats ✪ ✪

*N*amed for the famous naturalist, this heavily wooded trail meanders east to west, with north to south switchbacks, across nearly two miles of forest thick with sugar maples, ferns, and skunk cabbage, and in season, wildflowers, too. Parts of the path are lined with stone walls that once marked the boundaries of farms. The middle section, called Croton Woods, rises sharply along what once was the city's first water tunnel, and is the least-used part of the trail. Peaceful, yes, but I don't recommend this section as a solo excursion; experienced hikers know they should not go deep into the woods alone. The two access points are just north of the Riverdale Equestrian Centre near Broadway and West 254th Street, on the west side of the park, and at the Stockbridge Indian Memorial at Oneida Avenue and Van Cortlandt Park East, on the east side of the park. The memorial commemorates a band of Massachusetts Indians who were scouting for the Continental Army and slain here. There are also two wooded north to south trails—the Putnam Trail and the Old Croton Aqueduct Trail—wide enough and flat enough for hikers; both of these trails are primarily packed dirt tracks.

⌣ essentials

Van Cortlandt Park South (West 240th Street) to Parkway North and the border with Westchester County, between Broadway and Jerome Avenue and Van Cortlandt Park East; Bronx 10471

Friends of Van Cortlandt Park: (718) 601-1553; Urban Park Rangers: (718) 548-0912

nycgovparks.org/parks/vancortlandtpark or vancortlandt.org

Free admission

Open daily, 6 a.m.–1 a.m.

By subway: 1 to 242nd Street (last stop), then Bx9; 4 to Woodlawn Avenue (last stop), then Bx34 bus. **By bus:** Bx9 along Broadway (western edge of park); Bx16, 31, or 34 (eastern edge of park).

peaceful place 71

LINDEN TERRACE, FORT TRYON PARK
Washington Heights, Northern Manhattan

CATEGORY ⌣ parks & gardens ✪ ✪

*O*f all the appealing aspects of Fort Tryon Park, Linden Terrace wins my vote as the most relaxing spot. Dozens of towering trees frame the view across the Hudson River to New Jersey's Palisades cliffs, with lots of old-fashioned wood-slat park seating that invites lingering among the lindens. A plaque honors the Maryland and Virginia regiments who defended this ground in 1776 against the British, who renamed the outpost after the last British governor of Colonial New York City. Adjoining the terrace is the lush and charming Heather Garden, primarily a destination for strolling. And how pleasant that is any time of year, particularly from spring to fall when yellow and lavender heather fills the landscape.

⌣ essentials

✉	Broadway to Hudson River, between Riverside Drive and West 192nd Street, Manhattan 10040
☎	(212) 795-1388
🌐	nycgovparks.org/parks/forttryonpark
$	Free admission
🕐	Open daily, 5 a.m.–1 a.m.
🚍	**By subway:** A to 190th Street or Dyckman Street. **By bus:** M4 to the Cloisters, in Fort Tryon Park; M98 to 193rd Street.

peaceful place 72

LITTLE RED LIGHTHOUSE, FORT WASHINGTON PARK
Washington Heights, Northern Manhattan

CATEGORY ∿ scenic vistas ✪ ✪ ✪

*O*K, the official name is Jeffreys Hook Lighthouse, but New Yorkers never call it that. Nor did author Hildegarde H. Swift in her 1942 children's book *The Little Red Lighthouse and the Great Gray Bridge.* That classic encourages readers to "see for yourself," and you should. Manhattan's only remaining lighthouse was built in 1920 and remained in operation until 1947. The lighthouse "hero" of the book anchors the eastern side of the great, gray George Washington Bridge, which is almost directly overhead, all but hiding it from view. The site is rarely crowded because getting to it is so difficult. But the wonderful vistas up and down the Hudson River justify the effort. Remember to pack binoculars for bird-watching, and bring a picnic lunch. The Urban Park Rangers, from New York's Department of Parks & Recreation, provide tours from spring to fall about once a month.

∿ essentials

▤   Fort Washington Park, Riverside Drive at West 178th Street, Manhattan 10034

✆   (212) 304-2365

🌐   historichousetrust.org and nycgovparks.org/parks/fortwashingtonpark

$ Free admission

🕐   Call for lighthouse tour schedule. Park: open daily, 6 a.m.–1 a.m.

🚇   **By subway:** A to 181st Street; walk west to Lafayette Place; take steps, footbridge, and footpath over highway down to park and south to lighthouse.

peaceful place 73

LOBBY LOUNGE, MANDARIN ORIENTAL HOTEL
Upper Manhattan

CATEGORY ↵ quiet tables ✪ ✪

*S*itting in this 35th-floor sky lobby makes me feel like a bird soaring above the treetops of Central Park, just across the street. I like to take the elevator to the 36th floor, so I can float down the grand curved staircase and enjoy the view unfolding with each step. The lounge is especially calm in winter, when the park is cloaked in white after a snowstorm, and in spring, when the world is turning green. The view includes the statue of Christopher Columbus in the eponymous Columbus Circle. Beverages here are pricey, since this is a five-star hotel.

✈ essentials

≡ 80 Columbus Circle (at 60th Street), Manhattan 10023

☎ (212) 805-8876

🌐 mandarinoriental.com/newyork

$ Free admission

🕐 Monday–Thursday, 8 a.m.–11:30 p.m.; Friday–Saturday, 8 a.m.–12:30 a.m.; Sunday, noon–11:30 p.m.

🚌 **By subway:** 1, A, B, C, or D to 59th Street.
By bus: M5, 7, or 104 to 60th Street; M57 or 31 to Broadway.

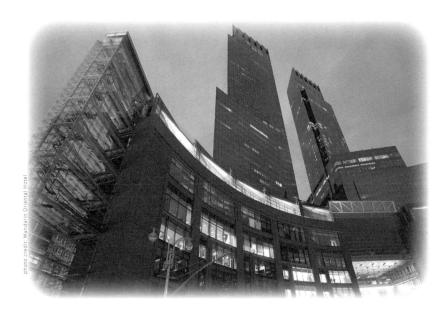

photo credit: Mandarin Oriental Hotel

Mandarin Oriental Hotel overlooks Columbus Circle.

peaceful place 74

LULLWATER AND PENINSULA TRAILS, PROSPECT PARK
Park Slope, Brooklyn

CATEGORY ⌣ outdoor habitats ✪ ✪ ✪

*T*wo well-marked walking trails fan out from behind the Prospect Park Boathouse. Both are looped paths that take 30 to 45 minutes each, at a leisurely pace. The Lullwater Trail offers some of the best bird-watching in the park, and you can find enthusiasts with binoculars at dawn and dusk, when the birds are most active. The feather aficionados scan the lush greenery for belted kingfishers in summer and red-tailed hawks in autumn. My favorite place when not hiking is the old-fashioned rustic shelter at the edge of the lake. When hiking, I prefer the Peninsula Trail, since it changes from open water to sometimes muddy wetlands to dry upland and back again. I wander past black cherry trees, shrubs that remind me of holiday holly, quacking ducks, and fish, including largemouth bass that lure the dreams of would-be fishermen, since fishing is catch-and-release only. Even though these trails are close to the boathouse, please be safe and sensible, and do not go alone here after dark.

⌣ essentials

⊟ Flatbush and Ocean avenues to Prospect Park Southwest, between Parkside Avenue and Prospect Park West; Brooklyn 11215

📞 (718) 287-3400   ⊕ prospectpark.org $ Free admission

🕐 Open daily, 5 a.m.–1 a.m.

🚇 **By subway:** Q, S, or B to Prospect Park; 2 or 3 to Eastern Parkway, or Q to Parkside Avenue. **By bus:** B69 or B75 to Prospect Park West and Ninth Street; B68 to Prospect Park West and 15th Street.

peaceful place 75

MADISON SQUARE PARK
Midtown Manhattan

CATEGORY ✌ parks & gardens ✪ ✪ ✪

*N*amed for the city's first Madison Square Garden that once stood here—replaced by one on 50th Street and Eighth Avenue, which was replaced by the current one over Penn Station at Eighth Avenue—the park stands in an eclectic neighborhood. The area has morphed from luxury residences in the 1800s to offices, many of which are now being turned back into expensive residential condos and lofts, with more new ones being built. The park has been upgraded with pretty plantings and paths, shaded by some of the largest-limbed trees you'll see in Manhattan. Plenty of benches, too, although you'll be sharing them with moms and nannies shepherding kids in the playground here. My favorite spot is close to 23rd Street, where I can gaze on the ornate splendor of the Flatiron Building, named for its triangular shape reminiscent of a clothing iron. Historical tidbit: The winds on this corner are such that construction workers on this palazzo-style skyscraper in the early 1900s were often able to catch a glimpse of a lady's ankle, which gave birth to the phrase "23 skiddoo" as the police tried to get onlookers to move along, or convince construction workers to get back to work.

✌ essentials

⌐	23rd to 26th streets between Fifth and Madison avenues, Manhattan 10010
☎	(212) 538-6667
🌐	nycgovparks.org/parks/madisonsquarepark or madisonsquarepark.org
$	Free admission ① Open daily, 7 a.m.–11 p.m.
🚌	**By subway:** 6, W, or R to 23rd Street. On weekends, take the N. **By bus:** M23 to Fifth or Madison avenues; M1, 2, 3, 5 to 23rd Street.

peaceful place 76

METROPOLITAN MUSEUM OF ART (selected rooms)
Upper East Side, Upper Manhattan

CATEGORY ⌣⁚ museums & galleries ✪ ✪ ✪

*S*imply one of the world's top art museums, it sprawls across four city blocks
at the edge of Central Park. The museum's size means that it shelters myriad
niches for those seeking a peaceful spot. My favorites are in the gallery housing Claude
Monet's *Morning on the Seine Near Giverny* and *Rouen Cathedral: The Portal (Sunlight)* paintings, and Georges Seurat's *Study for "A Sunday on La Grande Jatte."* I like to walk back and
forth to see how the brushstrokes change with distance. Also, I love wandering through
the Egyptian wing's Temple of Dendur, with its slanted wall of glass bathing the ancient
stones with delicious light and shadows. But never aim for serenity here on weekends,
when the museum is most crowded with a cacophony of visitors from around the world.
Other places in this sprawling museum that are least crowded include the Asian galleries
and the soaring spaces housing ancient Greek and Roman statuary.

⌣⁚ essentials

≡ᵈ   1000 Fifth Avenue (at 82nd Street), Manhattan 10028

✆   (212) 535-7710   ⊕ metmuseum.org

$ Adults $20; seniors $15; students $10; free for members, children under age 12 accompanied by an adult, and New York City public school students

🕐   Tuesday–Thursday, 9:30 a.m.–5:30 p.m.; Friday–Saturday, 9:30 a.m.–9 p.m.;
Sunday, 9:30 a.m.–5:30 p.m.

🚌   **By subway from the East Side of Manhattan:** 4, 5, or 6 to 86th Street, then walk three
blocks west to Fifth Avenue. **By bus:** M1, 2, 3, or 4 to 82nd Street. **By subway from the
West Side of Manhattan:** 1 to 86th Street, then the M86 bus across Central Park to
Fifth Avenue; or C to 81st Street, then the M79 bus across Central Park to Fifth Avenue.

peaceful place 77

MORGAN LIBRARY AND MUSEUM

Midtown Manhattan

CATEGORY ⌇ museums & galleries ✪ ✪ ✪

lease don't ask me which spot in this soaring, elegant place is my favorite. Sometimes I prefer the private study of John Pierpont Morgan, with its rich red silk damask walls hung with Italian Renaissance art. Other times, I head straight for Mr. Morgan's library, containing three stories of books from the 1400s to 1900s, where I will stand respectfully in front of the glass case holding a 1455 Gutenberg Bible, the first

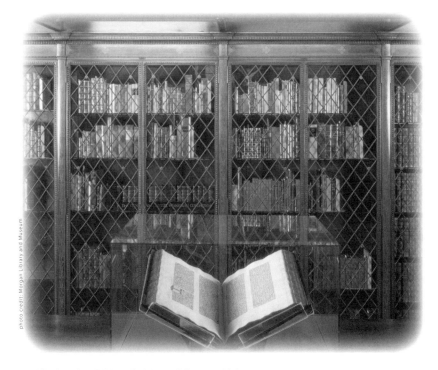

The Gutenberg Bible at the Morgan Library and Museum

substantial book published with movable type. I also like to sit on the bench in front of the library's massive fireplace to appreciate the ceiling, with images of zodiac signs and people reading books. Or I'll hang out in the large marble lobby between the two rooms, so I can look right and left at them both. In 2006, a modern addition to the Morgan opened and offers additional gallery space for rotating exhibits that almost always focus on a single author and his or her books. There's also a cafe in the glass-enclosed central court, where you can sit undisturbed before or after lunchtime.

✌ essentials

⌨	225 Madison Avenue (at 36th Street), Manhattan 10016
☎	(212) 685-0008 🌐 themorgan.org
$	Adults $12; seniors and students $8; free for members and children under age 12 accompanied by an adult
🕐	Open Tuesday–Thursday, 10:30 a.m.–5 p.m.; Friday, 10:30 a.m.–9 p.m.; Saturday, 10 a.m.–6 p.m.; Sunday, 11 a.m.–6 p.m.
🚍	By subway: 4, 5, 6, or 7 to 42nd Street/Grand Central Station; 6 to 33rd Street; B, D, F, or Q to 42nd Street. By bus: M34, 42, or 104 to Madison Avenue; M1, 2, 3, 4, or 5 to 36th Street.

peaceful place 78

MOSES MOUNTAIN, S. I. GREENBELT
Todt Hill, Staten Island

CATEGORY ◡ outdoor habitats ✪ ✪

*W*hen you come here, you will not be the first to exclaim, "I can't believe I'm in New York City!" The 360-degree panorama that greets you at the top of Moses Mountain is surprisingly pristine. Except for a few buildings poking through the trees, the view is exclusively of the undulating hills of Staten Island, including Todt Hill, the highest point on the Atlantic seaboard between southern Maine and Florida. About halfway up, look for a rock with mysterious carvings, thought to be Cyrillic. My favorite time of year here is fall, when the air is crisp, the maples and elms are at their multicolored peak, and the berries on the sumac trees turn golden in the sunshine. It's a mini vacation for the eyes and the soul, and ironic that the overlook is named for New York City's so-called master builder, Robert F. Moses, who almost destroyed the place in the 1960s to build a highway. This is really a mountain of rock blasted to make way for a highway and then dumped here.

◡ essentials

⌷ Manor Road and Rockland Avenue, Staten Island 10306

☏ (718) 351-3450   ⊕ sigreenbelt.org $ Free admission

⏱ Trails: open daily, sunrise to sunset

🚌 **By bus:** From the Staten Island Ferry Terminal, take bus S74 to Rockland Avenue, then transfer to the S54 or S57 to Manor Road.

peaceful place 79

MOUNT VERNON HOTEL MUSEUM AND GARDEN
Upper East Side, Upper Manhattan

CATEGORY ✧ historic sites ❂ ❂

he multipurpose name denotes that in the early 1800s, this was a hotel—
a country escape for residents of a city that extended barely to what is now
14th Street. It's also one of the oldest buildings in New York City, dating from 1799
when it was built as a carriage house for the 23-acre estate of the daughter and son-in-
law of John and Abigail Adams. Wander through a Colonial and Victorian time warp of
elegant furnishings that speak to a genteel way of life and a slower pace than we know
now. Ladies would never have been allowed in the Gentlemen's Tavern Room back then,
but these days I like to sit there and browse through one of the historic newspapers to
contemplate how much has changed—including newspapers themselves. The backyard
garden and its small terrace together create just one more surprising oasis in the middle
of Manhattan. The area is infused with lush plantings and benches. And after a period
of relaxation, busy Bloomingdale's lies only a couple of blocks away.

✧ essentials

▤ 421 East 61st Street (between First and York avenues), Manhattan 10065

☏ (212) 838-6678   ✈ mvhm.org

$ Adults $8; seniors and students $7; free for members and children under age 12

☽ Tuesday–Sunday, 11 a.m.–4 p.m. (last tour at 3:30 p.m.); closed in August

🚊 **By subway:** 4, 5, 6, N, or R to Lexington Avenue/59th Street; F to 63rd Street.
By bus: M31 or 57 to First Avenue; M15 to 61st Street.

peaceful place 80

MUSEUM OF JEWISH HERITAGE:
A LIVING MEMORIAL TO THE HOLOCAUST

Lower Manhattan

CATEGORY ∿ museums & galleries ✪ ✪ ✪

*O*f course the exhibits relating to the Holocaust are disturbing, but there are peaceful places here, too. The third floor is all about spiritual and religious renewal. The video snippets of music and star turns by composer Leonard Bernstein, entertainer Mel Brooks, comedian Harpo Marx, musician Benny Goodman, comedian Milton Berle, sculptor Louise Nevelson, fashion photographer Richard Avedon, and other notable people always make me smile. The most contemplative, Zen-like spot is the outdoor Garden of Stones, overlooking the Hudson. It is strewn with 18 huge, smooth boulders, each with a hole planted with a tiny sapling. It is easy to sit on one of the benches, listening to the muffled harbor sounds in the distance, and lose all sense of time while you contemplate the tenacity and fragility of life. The museum is least crowded on Friday afternoons.

∿ essentials

- ⬛ 36 Battery Place, Manhattan 10280

- ✆ (646) 437-4200   ✪ mjhnyc.org

- $ Adults $12; seniors $10; students $7; free on Wednesdays 4 p.m.–8 p.m. and for children under age 12

- 🕐 Open Sunday–Tuesday and Thursday, 10 a.m.–5:45 p.m.; Wednesday, 10 a.m.–8 p.m.; Friday, 10 a.m.–5 p.m. (during Daylight Saving Time), 10 a.m.–3 p.m. (Eastern Standard Time); the eve of Jewish holidays until 3 p.m.

- 🚌 **By subway:** 4 or 5 to Bowling Green; W or R to Whitehall; 1 to South Ferry; J, M, or Z to Broad Street. **By bus:** M1, 6, 9, 15, or 20 to Battery Place.

peaceful place 81

NATIONAL ARTS CLUB
Gramercy Park, Lower Manhattan

CATEGORY ⌣ museums & galleries ✪

*Y*ou don't have to be a member of the club to enjoy the art galleries, nor to delight in the grand carpeted, carved-wood Victorian staircase that takes you to the second-floor Grand Gallery. This is another secret spot few non-members know about, so it's always a nearly empty hideaway, just steps from famous Gramercy Park. The building itself is both a National Historic Landmark and a New York City Landmark, designed in part by Calvert Vaux, one of the creators of Central Park. Exhibits change every couple of weeks and rotate among paintings, photography, and other art forms. Be sure to call first, since the club is closed regularly for private events. Current members include actors Robert Redford and Dennis Hopper; past members have included photographer Alfred Stieglitz and western art sculptor Frederic Remington.

⌣ essentials

⊟   15 Gramercy Park South, Manhattan 10003

☎   (212) 475-3424   🌐   nationalartsclub.org

$ Free admission (business casual dress code)

🕐   Monday–Friday, 10 a.m.–5 p.m. (call ahead as private events may close galleries)

🚌   **By subway:** 4, 5, 6, or L to 14th Street/Union Square.
By bus: M101, 102, or 103 to 18th Street; M9 or 14 to Third Avenue.

peaceful place 82

NEW YORK PUBLIC LIBRARY, STEPHEN A. SCHWARZMAN BUILDING

Midtown Manhattan

CATEGORY ∿ reading rooms ✪ ✪ ✪

*E*verybody knows the massive, ornate Main Reading Room of the main branch from such movies as *Spider-Man* and *Breakfast at Tiffany's*, plus any number of TV shows set in Manhattan. Most certainly, it is a pleasant respite when there's no film crew shouting, "Quiet on the set." In all fairness, any such filming inside is done overnight, when the library is closed. Officially named the Deborah, Jonathan F. P., Samuel

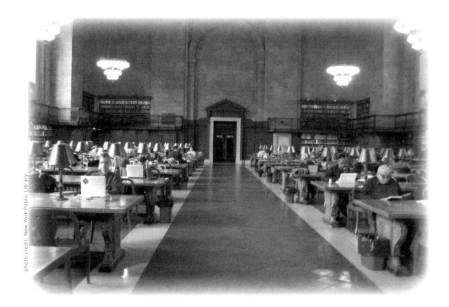

Main reading room of the New York Public Library on Fifth Avenue

Priest, and Adam R. Rose Main Reading Room, Room 315 is its common designation. So grand—at roughly two city blocks in length—it is divided in half, and its two-story height muffles sound better than earplugs.

The North Hall, on the right side of the entrance, is the quieter half, especially at the far end, farthest from the librarian's desk. Regardless, head for the South Hall, and keep walking down the corridor, past the people glued to public access computers, to the double doors of Room 300. This is the Art and Architecture room, a mini version of the main rooms, with the same massive wooden tables and reading lamps. Add to the experience by asking the librarian for a book about the Beaux Arts architecture of the building you are in. Or, avoid the upstairs rooms entirely and head for the Local History and Genealogy room (number 121) or the Current Periodicals room (number 108) on the main floor.

And remember to wave goodbye to Patience and Fortitude when you leave: Those are the two stone lions that famously guard the building, which was recently renamed the Stephen A. Schwarzman Building to recognize the Wall Street tycoon who donated an impressive $100 million to expand and modernize the New York Public Library system, including this landmark 1911 building.

⌣ essentials

▭   Fifth Avenue at 42nd Street, Manhattan 10018

☎   (917) 275-6975   🌐 nypl.org $ Free admission

🕐   Open Monday, Thursday–Saturday, 11 a.m.–6 p.m.; Tuesday–Wednesday,
      10 a.m.–9 pm; Sunday, 1 p.m.–5 p.m. (All rooms not open on Sundays.)

🚌   **By subway:** 1, 2, or 3 to 42nd Street/Broadway; 7 to Fifth Avenue; 4, 5, or 6 to Grand
      Central; D, B, or F to 42nd Street/Sixth Avenue.
      By bus: M1, M2, M3, M4, M5, M6, M7, M42, M104, or Q32 to 42nd Street/
      Fifth Avenue.

peaceful place 83

NEW YORK STATE SUPREME COURT, CIVIL BRANCH, NEW YORK COUNTY

Lower Manhattan

CATEGORY ↝ historic sites ✪

*Y*ou've watched actors rushing up and down the block-wide steps of this building in dozens of *Law and Order* episodes and in such movies as *The Godfather* and the classic 1947 *Miracle on 34th Street*. Even when cameras go inside, they fail to capture the grandeur of the arched entrance and huge domed rotunda, covered with a mural that reminds me of the Sistine Chapel in its scope and style. The painted dome

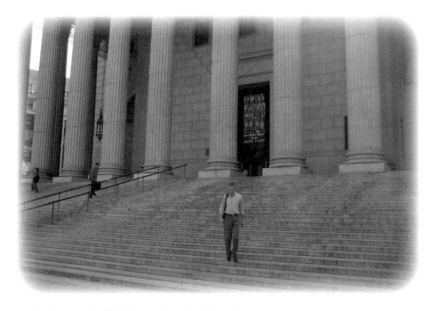

Grand entrance familiar from movies and television shows

depicts the history of law, from Byzantine to American, represented by figures including an Egyptian pharaoh, a Roman emperor, Moses, George Washington, and Abraham Lincoln. I actually don't mind the pain in my neck from looking up, or the slightly dizzy feeling I get from turning around on the equally grand marble floor, inlaid with all the astrological signs in bronze. The best times for an introspective visit are mid-morning and mid-afternoon, when court is in session and neither lawyers, plaintiffs, or court staff are rushing through the hall.

⌣ essentials

⌷   60 Centre Street, Manhattan 10007

🕐   (646) 386-3600

🌐   courts.state.ny.us

$ Free admission

🕐   Open Monday–Friday, 9 a.m.–5 p.m.

🚌   **By subway:** 4, 5, 6, J, or M to Chambers Street/Brooklyn Bridge;
     A, C, or E to Chambers Street; R or N to Canal Street.
     By bus: M1, 15, or 22 to Foley Square; M6 to City Hall.

peaceful place 84

ONASSIS CULTURAL CENTER
Midtown Manhattan

CATEGORY ⌣ museums & galleries ✪ ✪ ✪

*T*he guards usually outnumber the visitors at this hidden treasure, one of Midtown's least known and visited museum spaces. That makes the Onassis Cultural Center a lovely spot any time for communing with the gods and goddesses of ancient Greece, and for viewing the ancient pottery and other artifacts. Exhibits often include pieces on loan from cultural icons such as the State Hermitage Museum in St. Petersburg, Russia. Located in the Olympic Tower, built by Greek shipping tycoon Aristotle Onassis, the center is managed by an Onassis foundation. To get to the center, you'll have a pleasant stroll through the tower's atrium, which—except at the beginning and end of the workday—is itself peaceful. Copies of Greek friezes line the atrium, and you can enjoy them from the cluster of tables and chairs grouped beneath the skylight. Order a coffee from the tiny snack bar and relax.

⌣ essentials

   ✉   645 Fifth Avenue (between 51st and 52nd streets), Manhattan 10022

   ☎   (212) 486-4448   🌐 onassisusa.org $ Free admission

   🕐   Open Monday–Saturday, 10 a.m.–6 p.m.

   🚍   **By subway:** B, D, or F to 47th-50th Street/Rockefeller Center;
             6 to 51st Street/Lexington Avenue.
             By bus: M1, 2, 3, 4, 5, 6, or 7 to 50th Street; M27 or M50 to Fifth Avenue.

peaceful place 85

ORCHARD BEACH, PELHAM BAY PARK
East Bronx

CATEGORY ⌣ outdoor habitats ✪

*S*and and water, yes; surf, no, but that should not stop you from enjoying this crescent-shaped beach bordering Long Island Sound. You can escape the dueling boom boxes blasting salsa and hip-hop by heading to Quiet Zone sections 1, 2, and 3 to the far left of the main entrance. From Memorial Day to Labor Day weekends, there is no bicycle riding on the mile-long broad stone promenade. My spot of choice, though, is on the far side of the rock jetty at the end of Section 1, which opens on an enormous

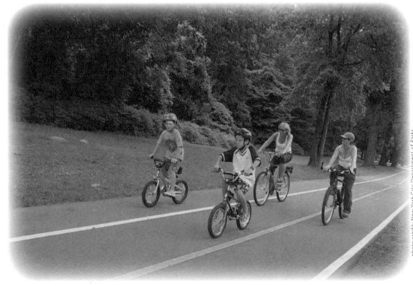

photo credit: New York City Department of Parks & Recreation, Malcolm Pinckney

One of many dedicated bicycle paths in Pelham Bay Park

rock "plaza" partly covered by moss and dried seaweed. Even on a crowded holiday weekend, just a few fishermen and picnickers are here parked under the shade of their umbrellas, and it's quiet enough to hear the water lapping gently against the rocky shore. Orchard Beach is part of sprawling Pelham Bay Park, the city's largest, whose nearly 2,800-acre expanse is three times the size of Manhattan's Central Park, which does not have 13 miles of saltwater shoreline, either.

⌣ essentials

⌨ Pelham Parkway East and Long Island Sound, within Pelham Bay Park; Bronx 10464

☎ (718) 430-1890

🌐 nycgovparks.org/parks/orchardbeach

$ Free admission

🕐 Open daily, 10 a.m.–6 p.m.

🚍 **By subway:** 6 to Pelham Bay Park (last stop), then connect to Bx29 or 52 bus. In summer, Bx5 and 12 serve the beach entrance; in winter, take Bx29 to the City Island Circle and walk approximately one mile to the beach.

peaceful place 86

PALEY PARK
Midtown Manhattan

CATEGORY ⌣ urban surprises ✪ ✪

*W*hen New York City's first so-called vest-pocket park entered the vocabulary in the 1960s, the idea was revolutionary. Until then, spaces between skyscrapers were ignored cavities of air. Paley Park changed all that, and it remains one of the best among the now-surprising number of tiny urban retreats. Its recycling waterfall wall blocks out street noise, the honey locust trees provide shade, and open-lattice chairs and tables enhance the feeling of light and space. A snack bar serves refreshments. Just

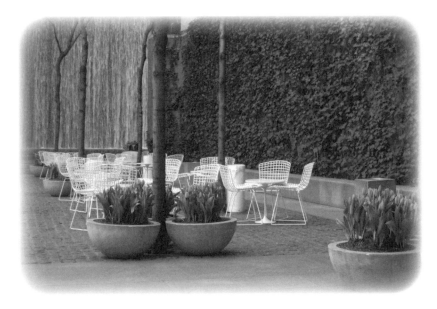

Paley Park invites lingering.

avoid lunchtime, when office workers rule. The park is named for the father of William S. Paley; William was one of the founders of CBS and, with his socialite wife, Babe Paley, a prominent philanthropist. Paley also started the Paley Center for Media museum a couple of blocks away—25 West 52nd Street, 10019, (212) 621-6600, paleycenter.org. There, you can watch historic videos of Edward R. Murrow, Walter Cronkite, and the *Apollo 11* moon landing—when you are ready for some excitement, that is.

⌣ essentials

⊡ 5 East 53rd Street (between Madison and Fifth avenues), Manhattan 10022

📞 No phone

🌐 No Web site

$ Free admission

🕐 Open daily, sunrise to sunset

🚌 **By subway:** E to Fifth Avenue/53rd Street; 6 to 51st Street and Lexington Avenue. **By bus:** M1, 2, 3, or 4 to 53rd Street; M27 or M50 to Fifth Avenue.

peaceful place 87

PIER 45 AND PIER 46, HUDSON RIVER PARK
West Village, Lower Manhattan

CATEGORY ↙ scenic vistas ✪ ✪ ✪

hese rebuilt piers are popular with local residents for suntanning and socializing, but the ambience is different. Families gravitate to the artificial turf areas of Pier 46, but because Pier 45 is three times as long, you are more likely to find a private spot for enjoying the view and have the sense of being in the middle of the river. The park between the two piers is slightly elevated, which effectively separates it from the activity on the wide walkway, and even on the most glorious day, you can usually find an empty chair to reposition for the view of your choice. There's also a permanent food and beverage kiosk, plus clean public bathrooms.

↙ essentials

✉	West 10th Street to Perry Street at the Hudson River, Manhattan 10014
☏	(212) 627-2020
🌐	hudsonriverpark.org
$	Free admission
🕐	Open daily, sunrise to sunset
🚌	**By subway:** 1 to Christopher Street/Sheridan Square; A, B, C, D, E, or F to West Fourth Street, then the M8 bus to pier.

peaceful place 88

PLUNGE BAR AND LOUNGE, HOTEL GANSEVOORT
Meatpacking District, Lower Manhattan

CATEGORY ↙ quiet tables ⊛

*T*he 360-degree view at sunset is beyond description, and you might even catch a glimpse of one of the celebrities who stay at this chic boutique hotel. You don't have to be a hotel guest to enjoy the rooftop bar, the lounge, or the view, but you do need a guest key to jump into its pool. The outdoor bar has a retractable glass roof that can be covered when the weather causes goose bumps on bare fashionista skin, which is exactly the best time to find solace 14 floors above the "in" crowd at street

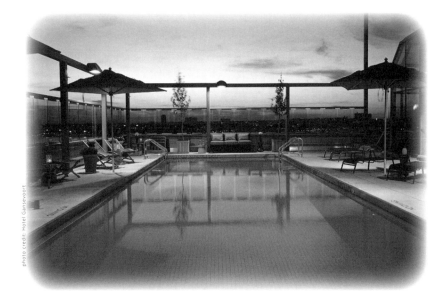

photo credit: Hotel Gansevoort

The Hotel Gansevoort rooftop overlooks the Hudson River.

level, even if you don't curl up with peaceful thoughts near the rooftop fireplace or the landscaped garden area. Of course the west side view is the Hudson River and the new High Line elevated park, but I actually prefer zoning out watching the ballet of cars and pedestrians on the northern side, overlooking 14th Street and Ninth Avenue. The rooftop is popular for corporate events, so phone before you go, to be sure it's open to the public when you want to visit.

⌣ essentials

▭ 18 Ninth Avenue, Manhattan 10014

✆ (212) 660-6736

✈ hotelgansevoort.com

$ Free admission; cost varies according to drink and menu selection

◔ Open daily, noon–4 a.m.

🚌 **By subway:** 1, 2, 3, A, C, or E to 14th Street, then either walk two to three long blocks, or take the M14 bus to Ninth Avenue and walk one block south to hotel.

peaceful place 89

POE COTTAGE, POE PARK

Fordham, Bronx

CATEGORY ⌣ historic sites ✪ ✪

*W*hen Edgar Allan Poe moved to this tiny wooden house in 1846, the area was called Fordham village. In those days, it was still a rural outpost, where he hoped the country air would help his wife's health, and he could write in silence. Poe wrote the classic poem "Annabel Lee" here, and lived here until his death in Baltimore in 1849. Though biographers tell us that Poe was tormented, his former home offers a spot of serenity. Today, this modest cottage sits pretty much ignored by the throbbing

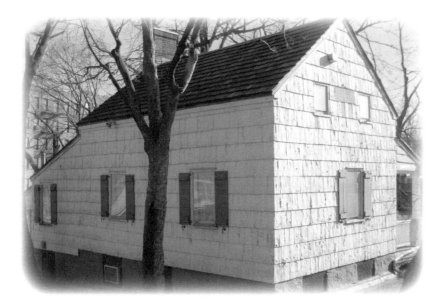

Edgar Allan Poe's simple wood-frame cottage

working-class neighborhood that surrounds it, at the northern edge of a small park in the middle of busy Grand Concourse. But it is definitely worth exploration and contemplation. In the three small rooms on the main floor, you can reflect on the author, consider what life was like in a simpler century, and measure how much quiet time it took to write in longhand with a quill pen.

⌣ essentials

🖃   Grand Concourse at East Kingsbridge Road, Poe Park, Bronx 10458

☎   (718) 881-8900   🌐   bronxhistoricalsociety.org/poecottage.html

$ Adults $5; seniors, students, and children $3

🕓   Open Monday–Friday, 9 a.m.–5 p.m.; Saturday, 10 a.m.–4 p.m.; Sunday, 1 p.m.–5 p.m.

🚋   **By subway:** D or 4 to Kingsbridge Road.
    By bus: Bx9, Bx22, or Bx28 to Kingsbridge Road/Grand Concourse.

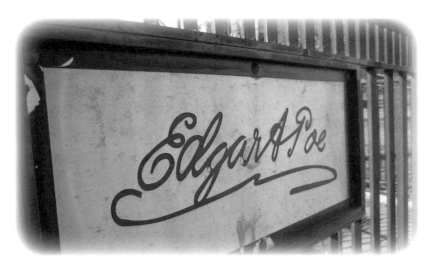

Replica of his signature at entrance to Poe Cottage

peaceful place 90

PROMENADE, RIVERSIDE PARK
Upper West Side, Upper Manhattan

CATEGORY ⌣ enchanting walks ✪ ✪ ✪

*P*ossibly because I've lived just a few blocks away from Riverside Park for several decades and have gotten to know it so well, my favorite part of the park is the Promenade. A broad boulevard from 79th to 92nd streets, it covers commuter train tracks, and its height offers a different viewpoint of the river. The northern end is marked by a lush community garden, lovingly tended by local residents with plantings that change seasonally. The southern end is marked by a memorial to Holocaust victims. There are abundant benches on both sides of the promenade facing the Hudson River, which sparkles between the trees. And there are lots of hilly, secluded paths off the Promenade where you can wander among mature cherry trees, lindens, and ginkgoes.

⌣ essentials

▤   Riverside Drive to Hudson River, 79th to 95th streets, Manhattan 10024

✆   (212) 408-0264

🐦   nycgovparks.org/parks/riversidepark

$ Free admission

🕐   Open daily, 6 a.m.–1 a.m., but not recommended after sunset

🚌   **By subway:** 1 or 2 to 79th to 96th streets.
      By bus: M104 or 5 to 79th to 96th streets, or M86 or 96 to Riverside Drive.

peaceful place 91

RADIANCE TEA HOUSE AND BOOKS
Midtown Manhattan

CATEGORY ↲ quiet tables ✪ ✪ ✪

*T*he golden honey tones of the wood floor and counters harmonize with the slightly darker wood of traditional carved wooden chairs and tables. This is a place to linger, restfully, over a pot of one of dozens of types of teas, including organics, with or without a plate or two of light Chinese dumplings, Japanese rice balls, Vietnamese summer rolls, and such. I like to wander to the other side of the shop to investigate the selection of handmade and painted tea sets for sale, leaf through books about tea, and check out the selection of loose teas to take home.

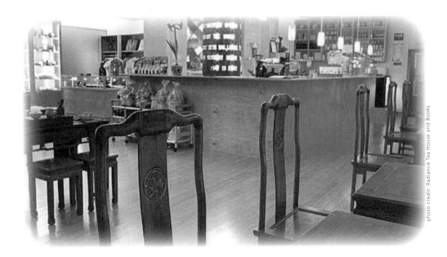

photo credit: Radiance Tea House and Books

Oriental calm at Radiance Tea House and Books

essentials

⌨ 158 West 55th Street (between Sixth and Seventh avenues), Manhattan 10019

☎ (212) 217-0442

🌐 radiancetea.com

$ Free admission; tea ceremony $35, requires reservation

🕐 Open Monday–Thursday, 10 a.m.–10 p.m.; Friday–Saturday, 10 a.m.–11 p.m.; Sunday, 11 a.m.–8 p.m.

🚌 **By subway:** F, N, R, Q, or W to 57th Street; E, B, or D to 53rd Street.
By bus: M5, 6, 7, or 104 to 55th Street.

peaceful place 92

RAMBLE, CENTRAL PARK
Upper Manhattan

CATEGORY ⌣ outdoor habitats ✪ ✪ ✪

*F*orever Wild is a designation shared by more than 50 sites considered to be ecologically significant in a program overseen by the New York City Department of Parks & Recreation. This hilly, overgrown 38-acre chunk of nature in the middle of Manhattan certainly lives up to its appellation. Spring through fall, tall leafy trees and vines almost entirely hide the surrounding skyline; in winter, the bare branches create a lacelike pattern stretching to the blue yonder.

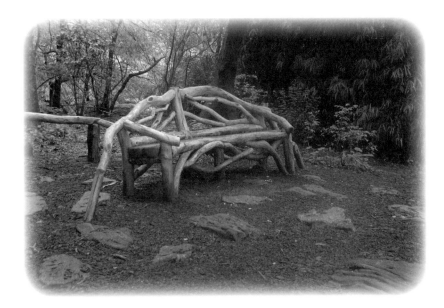

Rough-hewn bench in Central Park's Ramble

The Central Park Conservancy leads walking tours through the Ramble. But for your own private space, come here to walk for long stretches without encountering more than the occasional bird-watcher or dog walker. Central Park marks an important rest stop on the annual winged migration between South America and Canada, and because of its dense foliage, the Ramble is a favorite area for songbirds and other flying travelers. So do show up in the early morning, when the feathered ones are most active. I was lucky one fine spring day to prowl these sheltered paths with seasoned experts from the Audubon Society. We saw and heard more than 60 different species, including green herons, fluorescent blue indigo buntings, and a red-tailed hawk.

Because the Ramble's gravel and dirt paths, hills, and rocks pose rough riding for bicyclists and for toddlers in their strollers, this area remains a bucolic spot throughout the day—but, please, not after dark, as this is such a secluded site.

Most visitors enter the Ramble from the path just behind the Loeb Boathouse. Stay to the left when the path forks to walk along the Central Park lake. The path ends at the shoreline, where you'll reap a sweeping view of Bethesda Fountain and Plaza. But my vote for the best (and most romantic) spot in this part of Central Park is seen if you continue straight, where the clearing in the trees affords a glimpse of the Bow Bridge, named for its gentle Venice-like curve—and shown on this book's cover.

˘ː essentials

⌨   Mid-park between 73rd Street and the 79th Street Transverse, Manhattan 10021

✆   (212) 310-6600   ◉   centralparknyc.org $ Free admission

◔   Open daily, 6 a.m.–1 a.m., but absolutely not recommended before sunrise or after sunset

🚌   **By subway:** 1 to 79th Street/Broadway; B or C to 72nd or 80th streets.
By bus: M1, 2, 3, or 4 to 79th Street; M10 between 70th and 80th streets.

peaceful place 93

RAVINE, PROSPECT PARK
Park Slope, Brooklyn

CATEGORY ⌣ outdoor habitats ✪

*I*t should not surprise you that Prospect Park's Ravine is very similar to the rugged and overgrown terrain of the Ramble in Manhattan's Central Park. After all, both parks were designed by the same architect-landscaper team of Frederick Law Olmsted and Calvert Vaux. The Ravine is Brooklyn's only remaining forest, defined by a steep, narrow gorge lined with thick foliage that will make you think you are somewhere along the Adirondack Trail, hundreds of miles from Times Square, instead of a short walk from the nearest subway that will get you to 42nd Street in 30 minutes. Uneven paths that are unfriendly to children's strollers and bicycles, combined with its location in the center of the park, make this an underutilized yet lovely park area.

⌣ essentials

🖃 Flatbush and Ocean avenues to Prospect Park Southwest, between Parkside Avenue and Prospect Park West; Brooklyn 11215

☎ (718) 287-3400   🌐 prospectpark.org $ Free admission

🕒 Open daily, 5 a.m.–1 a.m., but not recommended before sunrise or after sunset

🚌 **By subway:** F to 15th Street/Prospect Park or Seventh Avenue;
2 or 3 to Grand Army Plaza; Q to Seventh Avenue.
By bus: B41 or B71 to Grand Army Plaza; B79 to Ninth Street/Prospect Park.

peaceful place 94

RIVERSIDE PARK

Upper West Side, Northern and Upper Manhattan

CATEGORY ⌣ scenic vistas ✪ ✪ ✪

*F*rom West 59th to West 126th streets, the green space along the Hudson is called Riverside Park, while the lower section, between the Battery and West 59th Street, is called Hudson River Park. Playgrounds ringing with the sounds of giggling children define some parts of Riverside, and enclosed dog runs, for those whose "children" have more than two feet, occupy other spaces. And benches line Riverside Park's broad walkway immediately along the river. I enjoy peering through the fence of the famous

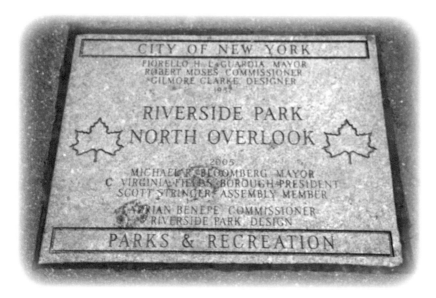

Riverside Park stretches for six miles along the Hudson River.

79th Street Boat Basin, pondering if I would enjoy living on one of the houseboats tied up here. My Riverside Park excursions always include the pier at 64th Street. It's more than 700 feet long—think 70-story building on its side jutting into the river—and it's never crowded, so there's always an empty bench where you can listen to the water lapping beneath you. To prepare for this lulling sensation, I like to come with a picnic: I recommend a bagel-and-lox sandwich, with a schmear of cream cheese, of course, from legendary (and not peaceful) Zabar's gourmet food store—2245 Broadway at 80th Street, 10024, (800) 697-6301, zabars.com. Feast while you watch the sunset, people fishing, or the tennis players on the clay courts at West 96th Street.

⌣ essentials

🖃	Riverside Drive to Hudson River, West 59th to West 126th streets, Manhattan 10115
☏	(212) 408-0264
🌐	nycgovparks.org/parks/riversidepark
$	Free admission
🕐	Open daily, 6 a.m.–1 a.m., but not recommended after sunset
🚇	**By subway:** 1 or 2 to any stop between 59th to 125th streets. **By bus:** M104 or 5 to 66th to 96th streets; M72, 86, or 96 to Riverside Drive.

peaceful place 95

ROBERT F. WAGNER JR. PARK
Lower Manhattan
CATEGORY ⌁ parks & gardens ✪

*N*amed after a popular three-term NYC mayor (1954–1965), this is both the northern extension of Battery Park and the southernmost park in the string of smaller parks along the Hudson River known collectively as the Greenway. It's favored more by local residents than tourists, so there's always room on the weathered teak benches, some of which are so wide that they are almost like a miniature boardwalk. The view extends to the cruise ship port in Bayonne, New Jersey, beyond the Statue of Liberty, and there's a small outdoor cafe in warm weather. The real treat, though, is to follow the waterside path north for about a half mile, past some trees and bucolic new landscaping.

⌁ essentials

⌑ Liberty Street and Pier A to the Hudson River, Manhattan 10004

📞 (212) 267-9700   🌐 bpcparks.org $ Free admission

🕐 Open daily, sunrise to sunset

🚇 **By subway:** 1 to South Ferry; 4 or 5 to Bowling Green; R or W to Whitehall Street.
By ferry: Staten Island Ferry to Battery Park.
By bus: M1, 6, 9, or 20 to Battery Park.

peaceful place 96

ROCKAWAY BEACH (streets above Beach 70th)
Rockaway, Queens

CATEGORY ↙ outdoor habitats ✪ ✪

*T*he last subway stop is at Beach 116th Street, so the farther you walk to higher street numbers, past the end of the boardwalk (leaving behind any food or other services) at Beach 126th Street, the emptier it gets, until it's just you, a local jogger or two, and the sandpipers. Beyond the end of the boardwalk, you'll move into a residential area with tree-lined streets and neat little front yards. The area has a definite suburban feel and has a peacefulness of its own, if you happen to like suburbia. The beach on this part of the Rockaway Peninsula is wider and more windswept than toward Far Rockaway, which adds appeal for me. But anywhere along this long finger of land, with Jamaica Bay on one side and the Atlantic Ocean on the other, is truly restorative.

↙ essentials

🖃 Atlantic Ocean, B90th to B135th streets, Queens 11693 and 11694

📞 (718) 318-4000

🌐 nycgovparks.org/parks/rockawaybeach

$ Free admission

🕐 Open daily, 6 a.m.–9 p.m.

🚌 **By subway:** A (Rockaway Park/B116th Street) to any stop after Broad Channel.

peaceful place 97

ROCKAWAY BEACH (streets below Beach 70th)
Rockaway, Queens
CATEGORY ⌣ outdoor habitats ✪ ✪

*W*hen the surf's up, the water is thick with foam and riders in black wet-suits. The designated ocean surfing area extends from Beach 67th to 69th streets and Beach 87th to 92nd streets, and it relaxes me to sit on the boardwalk or on the sand and watch the repetitive ballet of swoosh, dunk, and swim. The old-fashioned wooden boardwalk seems to run forever, and in some spots dunes and beach grass create the only canvas on this inland side for several blocks. In fact, each summer, in the Arverne neighborhood, volunteers and workers in the Forever Wild program managed by the New York City Department of Parks & Recreation cordon off wide strips of dunes between Beach 44th and 57th streets to protect breeding piping plovers, who nest here on their annual migration up and down the Atlantic Coast.

⌣ essentials

⌨ Atlantic Ocean, Beach Third to Beach 70th streets, Queens 11693

☎ (718) 318-4000

🌐 nycgovparks.org/parks/rockawaybeach

$ Free admission

🕐 Open daily, 6 a.m.–9 p.m.

🚇 **By subway:** A (Far Rockaway/Mott Avenue) to any stop after Broad Channel.

peaceful place 98

ROCKEFELLER CENTER CONCOURSE
Midtown Manhattan

CATEGORY ⌣ urban surprises ✪

*N*ew York natives like me know to avoid Rockefeller Center from the day the annual Christmas tree arrives until it's taken down to be turned into mulch for the city's parks and gardens. It's simply too crowded here during the holidays, during the peak tourist summer months, and also on early weekday mornings, when the NBC *Today* show takes its cameras outdoors into the plaza. Much quieter, any time, is the vast network of underground walkways linking the center's buildings. My favorite spot is called the Promenade, near the Sea Grill restaurant, where a couple of dozen tables and chairs are comfortable enough to stay for a while, but not all day. There's good lighting for reading or working on your laptop, but no outlets for plugging in. Avoid even this area during lunchtime, however, when it's packed with brown-bagging office workers who have discovered it.

While you are here, be sure to pick up a free guide at the visitor's desk at 30 Rock, the center's main building and home of NBC, to guide yourself on an introspective tour of the huge Art Deco murals that decorate the lobby. They depict science and industry, and it's interesting to contemplate how much things have changed in 80-ish years. Another tip: The benches outside, lining pedestrian-only Rockefeller Plaza, are a great place for people-watching, except when a special event—including a weekly warm-weather farmers' market—takes over.

⌁ essentials

🖃   47th to 51st streets between Fifth and Sixth avenues, Manhattan 10111

☎   (212) 632-3975

🌐   rockefellercenter.com

$ Free admission

🕐   Open daily, 7 a.m.–midnight

🚌   **By subway:** B, D, or F to 47th-50th Street/Rockefeller Center;
     1 to 50th Street; 6 to 51st Street; N, R, or W to 49th Street.
     By bus: M1, 2, 3, 4, 5, 6, or 7 to 50th Street; M27 or 50 to Fifth Avenue.

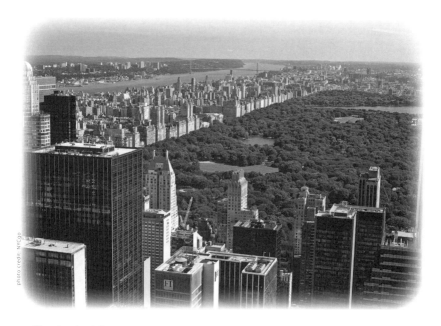

photo credit: NYCgo

View from 70th floor observatory at Rockefeller Center

peaceful place 99

ROOSEVELT ISLAND TRAMWAY

Roosevelt Island and Upper East Side, Upper Manhattan

CATEGORY ✎ scenic vistas ✪

I am a serious skier, so soaring above snow-capped mountains is something
I look forward to each winter. The scenery from this tram is no less wondrous—
the swirling waters of the East River and the dramatic landscape of Manhattan's
skyscrapers and bridges never fail to transport my spirits. And once I reach the island,
I love to visit the old lighthouse on the northern—car-free—end of the island. As for the
tram, however, you must choose your times wisely for a peaceful respite. Like the Staten
Island Ferry, the Roosevelt Island Tram is important transportation for workday commuters shuttling between the island and Manhattan's Upper East Side. It is one of the
few aerial commuter trams in North America, so for a calm outing, avoid early mornings
and late afternoons on weekdays.

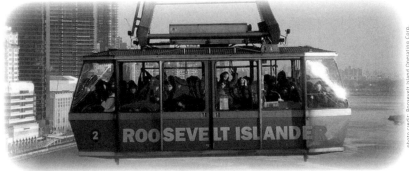

Roosevelt Island tram

⌣ essentials

▭ 591 Main Street, Roosevelt Island, Manhattan 10044

☎ (212) 832-4540   🌐 rioc.com

\$ The fare each way is \$2.25 (at press time), the same as that for NYC subway or bus lines.

🕐 Operates around the clock, though the schedule varies by day and time of day.

🚌 **By subway from Manhattan:** 4, 5, N, R, or W to Lexington Avenue/59th Street (Manhattan) and walk east to take the tram at Second Avenue and 59th Street. **By bus:** Q32, M31, or M57 to Lexington Avenue/59th Street. **By subway from Queens:** F to Roosevelt Island; N, 7, or W to Queensboro Plaza, then Q102 bus to Roosevelt Island.

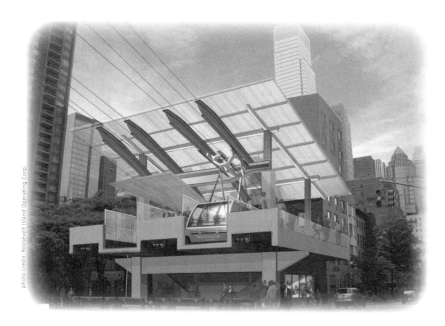

photo credit: Roosevelt Island Operating Corp.

Train station at 59th Street and Second Avenue

peaceful place 100

RUBIN MUSEUM OF ART
Chelsea, Lower Manhattan

CATEGORY ⌣ museums & galleries ✪ ✪ ✪

I n its previous life, this seven-story space was Barneys department store, but the only things you can buy now are in the gift shop, bookstore, and cafe. The seven floors of paintings, sculpture, textiles, and other artwork from the Himalayan region are just for admiring. There are multi-armed Shivas and gilded Buddhas in sizes from tabletop to monumental, plus watercolors, fabulously embroidered clothing, and more, from Tibet, Bhutan, Nepal, Mongolia, Iran, India, and other exotic locations. Some date from the 11th and 12th centuries, along with displays on more current social and cultural aspects of the regions. Most of the art here is from the collection of Shelly and Donald Rubin, who founded and funded the museum. Ascend the grand steel and marble staircase, by architect Andree Putnam, to view any one of the small, cozy anterooms of exhibits, and pause long enough before any of the many gods to be graced with their good karma. This museum is off the proverbial beaten track, even for Manhattanites, so it is rarely crowded except on Friday evenings, when admission is free and the otherwise quiet and pleasant lobby cafe turns into the loud and bustling K2 Lounge. Avoid the cafe at any time if it's peacefulness you are seeking, and go right upstairs to the galleries.

∵ essentials

150 West 17th Street (at Seventh Avenue), Manhattan 10011

(212) 620-5000

rmanyc.org

$ Adults $10; seniors, students, and neighbors $7; college students $2;
free for members and children under age 12

Open Monday and Thursday, 11 a.m.–5 p.m.; Wednesday, 11 a.m.–7 p.m.;
Friday, 11 a.m.–10 p.m.; Saturday–Sunday, 11 a.m.–6 p.m.

By subway: 1 to 18th Street; A, C, E, F, L, 1, 2, or 3 to 14th Street.
By bus: M6, 7, or 20 to Seventh Avenue/18th Street;
M5, 6, or 7 to Sixth Avenue/18th Street.

peaceful place 101

SCANDINAVIA HOUSE
Midtown Manhattan

CATEGORY ↲ museums & galleries ✪

*Y*ou don't have to be a descendant of ancestors from one of the Scandinavian countries to enjoy this place, which houses the offices of the American-Scandinavian Foundation. One floor hosts rotating exhibits featuring Scandinavian artists. Often the artwork is on loan from major museums and, while that draws crowds, Scandinavia House calms down after the first few days of such openings. The library and reading room also offer a quiet respite, especially since the iconic, streamlined Scandinavian table and chairs occupy space overlooking Park Avenue. The cafe in the atrium lobby has gotten too popular and too loud at lunchtime and after work, but is a welcome place at other times.

↲ essentials

[≡] 58 Park Avenue (at 38th Street), Manhattan 10016

ⓒ (212) 879-9779   🏵 scandinaviahouse.org $ Free admission

① Gallery: Tuesday–Saturday, noon–6 p.m. Library: Wednesday–Thursday and Saturday, noon–5 p.m. Cafe: Monday–Friday, 9 a.m.–10 p.m.; Saturday, 11 a.m.–10 p.m.; Sunday, 11 a.m.–5 p.m.

🚌 **By subway:** 4, 5, 6, 7, or S to 42nd Street/Grand Central Station; 6 to 33rd Street.
By bus: M34, 42, or 104 to Park Avenue; M1, 2, 3, 4, 5, 101, 102, or 103 to 36th Street.

peaceful place 102

SCHOMBURG CENTER FOR RESEARCH IN BLACK CULTURE

Harlem, Northern Manhattan

CATEGORY ⌣ reading rooms ✪ ✪ ✪

A modern arm of the New York Public Library, this center sits at one of the busiest intersections in Harlem. But open the heavy glass doors to enter an oasis. The cultural reservoir before you includes a research library, art gallery, and museum. Here, more than 10 million archived items document the history and ways of life of people of African descent worldwide. Galleries and art-embellished reading rooms occupy the first and second floors, where rotating exhibits focus on a particular theme, such as churches, music, or politics. One room overlooks a tiny outdoor courtyard and offers a welcoming respite. For thoughtful reflection, be sure to stop at the cosmogram on the ground floor just beyond the main entrance. A mosaic circle, it represents the Nile and other rivers associated with black history. Inscribed with the Mississippi River depiction are Langston Hughes refrains, such as, "My soul has grown deep like the rivers," from his poem "The Negro Speaks of Rivers."

⌣ essentials

📄 515 Malcolm X Boulevard (Lenox Avenue) at 135th Street, Manhattan 10037

📞 (212) 491-2200   🌐 nypl.org/research/sc $ Free admission

🕐 Monday–Wednesday, noon–8 p.m.; Thursday–Friday, 11 a.m.–6 p.m.; Saturday, 10 a.m.–5 p.m. (some rooms by appointment only)

🚌 **By subway:** 2 or 3 to 135th Street.
By bus: M7 or 102 to 135th Street; Bx33 to Malcolm X Boulevard.

peaceful place 103

SHORE PARKWAY PROMENADE
Bay Ridge, Brooklyn

CATEGORY ↝ outdoor habitats ✪ ✪ ✪

*M*ore than two miles of waterfront promenade are sprinkled with enough benches and vistas to provide a solo spot, even on a warm-weather weekend morning. You can easily ignore families taking a break from cycling and enjoy

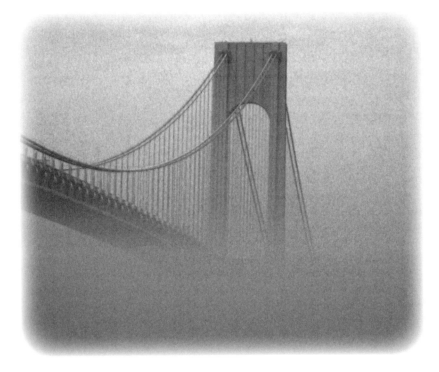

The Verrazano Bridge, lost in morning fog

small groups of tai chi practitioners in their silent, dancelike, slow-motion exercises. My favorite spot is almost under the Verrazano-Narrows Bridge, when it is clouded by fog and the Staten Island side is invisible in the distance. I am happily enthralled watching the towers and cables appear or disappear, depending on whether the fog is rolling in or out. Take that, you San Francisco and Golden Gate Bridge fans! My other favorite times are high and low tides, to watch another silent, slow-motion ballet, as massive cruise ships glide past, en route to or from their Hudson River or bay berths. The other key spot is the end of the pier at 69th Street for its provocative views of the Statue of Liberty and Lower Manhattan.

⌣ essentials

▣	Shore Road, 69th Street to Bay Parkway; Brooklyn 11209, 11228, and 11214
☎	(212) 639-6975
🌐	No Web site
$	Free admission
🕐	Open daily, sunrise to sunset
🚇	**By subway:** R to Bay Ridge Avenue. **By bus:** B1 to Bay Ridge and Fourth avenues.

peaceful place 104

SMITHSONIAN NATIONAL MUSEUM OF THE AMERICAN INDIAN, GEORGE GUSTAV HEYE CENTER
Lower Manhattan

CATEGORY ⌣ museums & galleries ✪

*T*he best time to visit this treasure trove of artifacts representing indigenous tribes and cultures from Alaska to Patagonia is weekday afternoons, after the school groups have left. I like to park myself on a bench in front of one of the intricately beaded buckskin dresses from the Plains Indians, to be soothed by their painstaking craftsmanship. Then I wander through rooms showcasing equally complicated basketry and carved jadeite from Mexico's Olmecs and Maya, and then on to the Hopi kachinas of U.S. Southwestern tribes. But my real secret spot is the small research library just off the front entrance. There, yet more priceless artifacts perch atop the bookcases and on the shelves, displayed similarly to the way you would show them in your own home. The museum is housed in a massive 1907 Beaux Arts edifice, the Alexander Hamilton U.S. Custom House, with ornate marble floors and columns and a rotunda that reminds me of the U.S. Capitol.

⌣ essentials

▤	One Bowling Green, at the north end of Battery Park, Manhattan 10004
☎	(212) 514-3700 ⊕ americanindian.si.edu $ Free admission
🕐	Open daily, 10 a.m.–5 p.m. (Thursdays to 8 p.m.)
🚌	**By subway:** 1 to South Ferry; 4 or 5 to Bowling Green; R or W to Whitehall Street; M, J, or Z to Broad Street. **By ferry:** Staten Island Ferry to Battery Park. **By bus:** M1, 6, or 15 to South Ferry.

peaceful place 105

SOCRATES SCULPTURE PARK
Long Island City, Queens
CATEGORY ☙ scenic vistas ⭐

*D*epending on your taste, the outdoor metal and mixed-media sculptures in this waterside park are either art or junk, but there's no disagreement on the view across sheltered Hallett's Cove to Roosevelt Island and Upper Manhattan. Get a picnic lunch from the take-out section of the giant Costco next door, and sit on the lawn inside a circle of recently planted young trees. Or choose one of the benches along the waterfront, where you will be charmed and calmed by the gentle lapping of the water. On Sundays from mid-May to September, the Long Island City Community Boathouse [(718) 228-9214, licboathouse.org] offers free kayaking off the small pier here.

☙ essentials

📧 32-01 Vernon Boulevard (at 31st Avenue), Queens 11106

📞 (718) 956-1819

🌐 socratessculpturepark.org

$ Free admission

🕐 Open daily, 10 a.m. to sunset

🚌 **By subway:** N or W to Broadway, and walk west on Broadway to park (about 15 minutes).

peaceful place 106

SOUTH BEACH AND MIDLAND BEACH
Staten Island

CATEGORY ↙ scenic vistas ✪ ✪

*W*hat could be better than a day at the beach with a view of Manhattan across the bay, and the soaring splendor of the Verrazano-Narrows Bridge? My favorite spot at these two connected beach areas is the northern edge of South Beach, closest to the bridge and at the end of the old-fashioned two-mile wooden boardwalk. That serves up a restorative combination of two of my favorite things— the beach and my hometown's skyline. There's plenty of sand, but no surf, since these adjoining beaches are in New York Harbor, not the Atlantic Ocean, so you'll be meditating on gentle ripples of tide instead of thundering foam, and the occasional cruise ship or tanker gliding by.

↙ essentials

✉	Father Capadanno Boulevard and Sand Lane, Staten Island 10301
✆	South Beach: (718) 816-6804; Midland Beach: (718) 987-0709
🌐	nycgovparks.org/parks/R046
$	Free admission
🕐	Open daily, sunrise to sunset (Swimming allowed Memorial Day weekend– Labor Day, 10 a.m.–6 p.m.)
🚌	**By bus:** From the Staten Island Ferry Terminal, take S51 to beach entrance.

peaceful place 107

ST. ANN AND THE HOLY TRINITY EPISCOPAL CHURCH

Brooklyn Heights, Brooklyn

CATEGORY ︙ spiritual enclaves ✪

*T*he organ at this Gothic Revival church is named for George Foster Peabody—founder of the prestigious Peabody Award for journalism—who worshiped here and financed the organ. There's a free recital at 1:10 p.m. every Wednesday on the historic full-throated instrument, and meditation each weekday from noon to 2 p.m. Another standout feature of this soot-stained 1844 church is its original stained-glass windows—64 of them, which are not visible from the street. Each window depicts a different biblical scene. Choose a pew in front of whichever window you pick as your favorite du jour, and let the magic of the colors and details calm your brain.

︙ essentials

▤	157 Montague Street (at Clinton Street), Brooklyn 11201
☎	(718) 875-6960
⊕	saintannandtheholytrinity.org
$	Free admission
◷	Open Monday–Friday, noon–2 p.m.; Sunday service, 11 a.m.
🚍	**By subway:** 2, 3, M, or R to Court Street; A, C, or F to Jay Street/Borough Hall.

peaceful place 108

STATEN ISLAND FERRY
Staten Island and Lower Manhattan

CATEGORY ⌣ scenic vistas ✪

A fleet of nine ferries makes the 25-minute trip every day, rain or shine— and it's free! And yes, it can be crowded, so you have to pick the right time. Since the 1700s, ferries have been transporting visitors and commuters between two of the world's most famous islands—Manhattan and Staten—and of course have appeared in countless movies and TV shows. So no surprise that the Staten Island Ferry is the third most-visited attraction in New York City, after the Statue of Liberty and the Empire State Building. So if people-watching puts you into a tranquil state of mind, here is the place to hang out: You can distinguish the commuters—they are the ones reading their newspapers, thumbing their BlackBerrys and iPhones, dozing, or otherwise ignoring the sweeping views.

But if it's views that lull you into a blissful frame of mind, just turn your gaze out to the Statue of Liberty, Ellis Island, the Lower Manhattan skyline, the graceful stretch of the Verrazano-Narrows Bridge, and skyscraper-size cruise ships heading to or from port on the Hudson River. When it's raining or cold and windy, I'll stay warm and cozy inside and watch the passing display through the windows. Otherwise, look for me on the top deck, taking deep, calming breaths of scenery scented with salt air. The ferry operates around the clock, so you can see the city framed by sunrise, sunset, or under sparkling nighttime lights. Just avoid morning and afternoon rush hours.

⌣ essentials

   Whitehall Ferry Terminal (South Ferry), 4 South Street, Manhattan 10004;
St. George Ferry Terminal, 1 Bay Street, St. George, Staten Island 10301

☎ (718) 876-8441   🌐 siferry.com $ Free admission

🕐 Operates daily, around the clock, either hourly or every half hour, depending on time of day and day of week

🚌 **By subway to Whitehall Terminal:** 1 to South Ferry; J, M, or Z to Broad Street; R or W to Whitehall Street; 4 or 5 to Bowling Green.
By bus to Whitehall Terminal: M1, 6, 9, or 15.
By bus to St. George Terminal: S40, 42, 44, 46, 48, 51, 52, 61, 62, 66, 67, 74, 76, 78, 81, 84, 90, 91, 92, 94, 96, or 98.
By rail to St. George Terminal: Staten Island Railway to St. George.

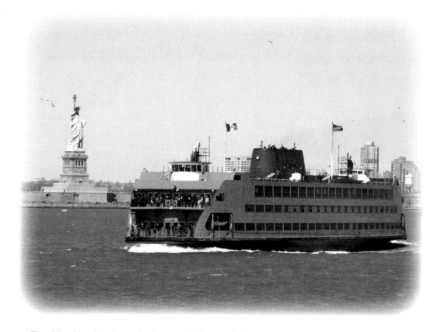

Two New York City icons: the Statue of Liberty and the Staten Island Ferry

peaceful place 109

STATEN ISLAND ZOO
West Brighton, Staten Island

CATEGORY ⌣ outdoor habitats ✪ ✪

anhattan's Central Park Zoo is easier to get to, and the sprawling Bronx Zoo is world-famous. Both, however, are usually crowded and not especially peaceful. This is the quiet alternative, partly because so many of its inhabitants are silent: Opened in 1936, the Staten Island Zoo has one of the largest collections of rattle-snakes in North America. They are housed in a sinuous building with a 100-foot-long faux snake skeleton hanging from the ceiling. If cold-blooded critters aren't your thing, outdoor areas are home to otters, cute furry meerkats, and red pandas that look more like raccoons than pandas. The Children's Zoo re-creates a barnyard setting, and ample tree-shaded walkways and benches lure you to sit and enjoy the antics of creatures both human and not.

⌣ essentials

614 Broadway, Staten Island 10310

(718) 442-3100   statenislandzoo.org

$ Adults $8; seniors $6; children ages 3–14 $5; free for children under age 3

Open daily, 10 a.m.–4:45 p.m.

By bus from the Staten Island Ferry terminal in St. George: Take the S48 bus to Forest Avenue and Broadway; walk left on Broadway to zoo entrance.
By bus from Brooklyn: Take the S53 bus from 95th Street and Fourth Avenue in Bay Ridge (near the BMT subway) to the zoo.

peaceful place 110

STEINBERG FAMILY SCULPTURE GARDEN, BROOKLYN MUSEUM

Prospect Heights, Brooklyn

CATEGORY ⌣ parks & gardens ❄ ❄

*P*riceless Greek and Roman sculptures dot this tree-bordered oasis squeezed between the Brooklyn Museum and its parking lot. Other pleasing visuals include huge copper vats and a 30-foot replica of the Statue of Liberty that was rescued from the top of Liberty Warehouse, near Lincoln Center. Flip a coin, or take your pick: Sit in an open, sunny plaza, or stroll to the tree-shaded half with old-fashioned park benches and semicircular stone slabs that ring the tall maples and oaks. And watch your step on the uneven brick walkways.

⌣ essentials

▭ 200 Eastern Parkway (behind the Brooklyn Museum), Brooklyn 11238

☎ (718) 638-5000

☛ brooklynmuseum.org

$ Free admission

⊙ Open Wednesday–Friday, 10 a.m.–5 p.m.; Saturday–Sunday, 11 a.m.–6 p.m. and to 11 p.m. on the first Saturday of each month

🚌 **By subway:** 2 or 3 to Eastern Parkway.
By bus: B71 to museum or B48 to Franklin Avenue and Eastern Parkway.

peaceful place 111

STEUBEN GLASS
Upper East Side, Upper Manhattan

CATEGORY ⌣ shops & services ✪ ✪ ✪

I have a love for the clarity and craftsmanship of handblown and hand-cut crystal, so the flagship Steuben store is an oasis of calm beauty for me. I head past the displays of beautiful, desirable bowls and goblets for sale to a circular staircase that descends to the museumlike exhibition area. Here you'll find three-masted schooners under full sail, breaching whales, New York City skyscrapers, galloping horses, and other exquisite creations suspended silently inside flawless crystal display cases, cushioned by black velvet and gleaming beneath pin-spot lighting. Walk around the protective cases to fully appreciate the details of the artisans' sparkling wonders. In this almost always empty gallery of the store, I find the crystal art inspiring, and time passes slowly while I linger.

⌣ essentials

✉   667 Madison Avenue (between 60th and 61st streets), Manhattan 10021

☎   (212) 752-1441   🌐 steuben.com

$ Free admission (but of course you are also free to purchase glassworks)

🕐   Monday–Saturday, 10 a.m.–6 p.m.

🚇   **By subway:** 4, 5, N, R, 6, or W to 59th Street/Lexington Avenue; 6 to 67th Street.
By bus: M1, 2, or 3 to 67th Street; M66 to Madison Avenue.

peaceful place 112

STONE STREET
Lower Manhattan

CATEGORY ↙ urban surprises ✪ ✪

*J*ust two blocks long, this narrow, cobblestoned street is reportedly the oldest paved street in Manhattan, and many of the buildings also date from the early 1800s. No traffic is permitted, and this charming little street is filled with picnic tables from its pubs, restaurants, and cafes. Some even supply the day's newspaper, and you can linger undisturbed with a beverage or two of your choice. Of course, lunchtime and Sunday brunch time are the most crowded times, which you will want to avoid.

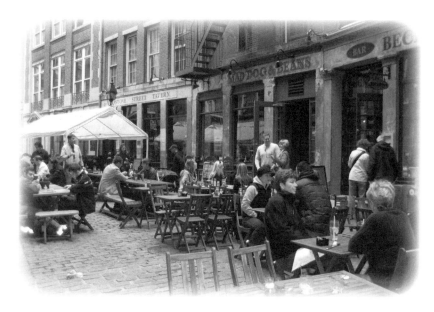

Cobblestones and cafe tables on Stone Street

✌ essentials

Between William Street and Coenties Alley, Manhattan 10004

No phone   No Web site $ Free admission

Open daily, 8 a.m.–2 a.m.

By subway: 2 or 3 to Wall Street; J, M, or Z to Broad Street; R or W to Whitehall/South Ferry.
By bus: M1, 6, 9, or 15 to William Street.

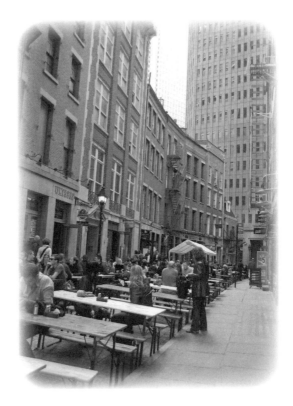

Historic Stone Street, steps from modern skyscrapers

peaceful place 113

ST. PAUL'S CHAPEL
Lower Manhattan

CATEGORY ⌣ spiritual enclaves ✪ ✪ ✪

*M*iraculously, the 1766 church and its small cemetery survived the September 11, 2001, attack that destroyed the World Trade Center and other buildings surrounding it. The chapel served as a 24-hour dormitory, cafeteria, and spiritual sanctuary to thousands of police, firefighters, and other volunteer responders from around the world. St. Paul's was a refuge over the months as they took breaks from searching through the rubble for remains of the victims. The heart-rending pile of their uniform badges will draw you to reflect in a corner a few steps from the roped-off pew where George Washington worshiped both as Revolutionary War general and first U.S. president. The benches in front of the chapel overlook the historic gravestone area, which is very parklike thanks to tall, stately trees. Just beyond lies the reconstruction of the World Trade Center site. Office workers tend not to sit here during the week, so weekdays are a better time to visit than weekends, when it's a popular tourist destination. To share this spot with like-minded souls, visit on Mondays and Thursdays for the free noontime concerts.

⌣ essentials
_____

▤ 209 Broadway (at Fulton Street), Manhattan 10007

✆ (212) 233-4164   ✈ saintpaulschapel.org $ Free admission

🕐 Open Monday–Saturday, 10 a.m.–6 p.m.; Sunday, 9 a.m.–4 p.m.

🚍 **By subway:** A, C, J, M, Z, 1, 2, 3, 4, or 5 to Fulton Street/Broadway-Nassau.
By bus: M1 or 6 to Fulton Street.

peaceful place 114

STRAND BOOKS
Union Square, Lower Manhattan

CATEGORY ⌣ shops & services ❶ ❶ ❶

*W*alk through the front door of what is known as the Strand, and you'll face more than 18 miles of packed shelves. All seem to call your name for browsing, wandering, contemplating, and escaping. Owners of this massive used-book store in New York City have been buying and reselling since 1927. The front of the store, with tables of cheap hard covers and paperbacks, is the most crowded—with books and people. So I advise you to go immediately to the stacks upstairs or to those in the basement. I usually leave a trail of breadcrumbs, Hansel and Gretel style, to find my way out again. Just kidding, but not kidding about wearing other than your best clothes here, since the Strand is not known for dusting.

⌣ essentials

▧   828 Broadway (at 12th Street), Manhattan 10003

℄   (212) 473-1452

🌐   strandbooks.com

$ Free admission

🕐   Monday–Saturday, 9:30 a.m.–10:30 p.m.; Sunday, 11 a.m.–10:30 p.m.
      Rare book room closes daily at 6:15 p.m.

🚌   By subway: N, R, Q, L, W, 4, 5, or 6 to Union Square.
      By bus: M1, 2, 3, 5, or 7 to Union Square.

STUYVESANT SQUARE PARK
Lower Manhattan

CATEGORY ↙ parks & gardens ❁ ❁

*O*nce part of Peter Stuyvesant's 17th-century farm, this four-block patch of seasonal flowers and grass serves today mostly as a shortcut between First and Third avenues, for those who know about it. Plenty of benches coax you to reflect, perhaps, on a passing squirrel or a delicate monarch butterfly. The square's famous—and decidedly private—neighbor, Gramercy Park, is closed to all who do not have a resident's key. I find it insulting to peer through the wrought-iron fence like a beggar, even though the plantings are gorgeous and sometimes I cannot help myself! However, Gramercy Park is notable for the landmark 19th-century town houses and mansions that border it, so after you enjoy their facades, go seat yourself in the sunshine of free and public Stuyvesant Square. Make time for lunch or dinner at Pete's Tavern a few blocks away— 129 East 18th Street, 10003, (212) 473-7676, petestavern.com. O. Henry was a tavern regular, and he wrote *The Gift of the Magi* in one of the burnished wooden booths. Ask your bartender or waiter which one—he or she will know. Perhaps your peaceful respite at Stuyvesant Square will have inspired you to pen a passage or two.

↙ essentials

▭ Rutherford Place to Nathan D. Perlman Place, Second Avenue between East 15th to East 17th streets; Manhattan 10003

✆ (212) 639-9675   🌐 nycgovparks.org/parks/M086 $ Free admission

🕑 Open daily, 6 a.m.–1 a.m.

🚍 **By subway:** 4, 5, 6, L, N, Q, R, or W to 14th Street/Union Square.
By bus: M14 to Second Avenue; M15 to 15th Street.

peaceful place 116

SUTTON PLACE PARK
Midtown Manhattan

CATEGORY ↝ urban surprises ✪ ✪ ✪

*I*t should come as no surprise that the residents of the multimillion-dollar apartments and town houses at this world-famous address don't want you to know about the small riverside park that's accessed from a hidden, unmarked spot. Ask where the entrance is, and you're likely to be met with a shrug and a Cheshire cat smile. But this little gem is just too good not to share. And, after all, it is a public park, not a private club for the genteel locals and their pampered pooches. So how do you find it? Beyond the opening in the retaining wall at the foot of 57th Street, a somewhat steep switchback ramp descends almost to the edge of the East River. Voilà! Here's how I spend my time in this tucked-away spot: watching the airborne Roosevelt Island tram seemingly float above and across the water, looking down and tracking the tiny whirlpools as they move with the East River current, and waving back at passengers chugging past on one of the Circle Line excursion boats. Ah, yes, life is good on Sutton Place.

↝ essentials

🖃   Sutton Place (between 56th and 57th streets at East River), Manhattan 10022

☏   (212) 639-9675   🕸 nycgovparks.org/parks/M108R $ Free admission

🕐   Open daily, 6 a.m.–1 a.m., but not recommended after sunset

🚌   **By subway:** 4, 5, or 6 to 59th Street.
    By bus: M57 or 31 to York Avenue; M15 to 57th Street.

peaceful place 117

TOP OF THE ROCK
Midtown Manhattan

CATEGORY ↙ scenic vistas ⭐

*T*he views are picture-postcard perfect from this 70th-floor observation deck. You'll gaze north across Central Park, west to the cruise ships berthed on the Hudson River, south to the Statue of Liberty, and southeast to the Brooklyn Bridge. The least crowded times are any day before 11 a.m., after 10 p.m., and also, surprisingly, at sunset. Now, that's just plain silly, because of course sunset is both enormously calming and undeniably romantic.

↙ essentials

⊟ 30 Rockefeller Plaza (entrance on 50th Street between Fifth and Sixth avenues), Manhattan 10012

☎ (212) 698-2000

🌐 topoftherocknyc.com

$ Adults $21; seniors $19; children ages 6–12 $14; free for children under age 5

🕐 Open daily, 8 a.m.–midnight (last elevator run is at 11 p.m.)

🚌 **By subway:** B, D, or F to 47th-50th Street/Rockefeller Center; 1 to 50th Street.
By bus: M1, 2, 3, 4, 5, 6, or 7 to 50th Street; M27 or M50 to Fifth Avenue.

peaceful place 118

TUDOR CITY GREENS
Midtown Manhattan

CATEGORY ↭ urban surprises ✪

lthough this is an enclave of private apartment buildings adjacent to the United Nations, two of the small landscaped areas between groups of buildings are public space. When you escape to this peaceful place, just behave as though you live and belong here, and you will be fine. To get here, climb the steps from busy 42nd Street to an instantly hushed world of shady trees and plantings that muffle street noise to a barely audible hum. Sometimes I choose a bench facing east for a view of the U. N. through the trees. Or I will pick a bench facing west for a peek of the Chrysler Building. But you can sit in any direction to enjoy the coats of arms and other froufrou on the Tudor-style architecture for which this 1920s complex was named. Avoid September through December, when the U.N. General Assembly is in session, or any time a high-profile official is speaking there, as then you would need to prove you live there to get through the security perimeter.

↭ essentials

⌷ East 41st to East 43rd streets (between First and Second avenues), Manhattan 10017

☎ (212) 949-6555   ☺ tudorcitygreens.org $ Free admission

☺ Open daily, sunrise to sunset

🚌 **By subway:** 4, 5, 6, or 7 to Grand Central Station.
By bus: M104, 42, 25, 27, or 50 to First Avenue; M15 or 16 to 42nd Street.

peaceful place 119

TWIN ISLANDS AND KAZIMIROFF NATURE TRAILS, ORCHARD BEACH AT PELHAM BAY PARK

East Bronx

CATEGORY ✎ outdoor habitats ✪ ✪

*B*oth trails are accessed near the Environmental Center, on the promenade at Section 2. The Twin Islands trail is a short loop that returns you to the center. Stay to the left to get on a dirt trail that rings a marshy area with a small sand beach populated by shorebirds including graceful egrets. It's much more peaceful than the paved path you'll be sharing with bicycles and baby strollers. And you're more likely to spot one of the resident ospreys from the woodsy dirt path. The Kazimiroff Nature Trails are two tree-shaded treks from the beach to the main access road, so they're a great way to arrive at the beach or leave it.

✎ essentials

✉ Pelham Parkway East and Long Island Sound, Environmental Center at Orchard Beach, within Pelham Bay Park; Bronx 10464

☎ (718) 885-3467

🌐 nycgovparks.org/parks/pelhambaypark

$ Free admission

🕐 Open daily, sunrise to sunset; Beach: 10 a.m.–6 p.m.

🚌 **By subway and bus:** 6 to Pelham Bay Park (last stop) and connect to bus Bx29 or 52. In summer, Bx5 and 12 serve the beach entrance; in winter, take Bx29 to the City Island Circle and walk approximately one mile to the beach.

peaceful place 120

230 FIFTH

Midtown Manhattan

CATEGORY ⌣ quiet tables ✪

*L*uckily, the palm trees and other greenery at this rooftop bar do not block the sight of the Empire State Building a few blocks away. The experience here ranges from tranquil and empty to packed and pumping, depending on day of week and time of year. Peacefulness seekers should simply avoid warm-weather visits, especially on weekends. Any other time, you can zone out on one of the comfy couches and stare at the vista in solitude. Whenever the thermometer dips below 55, the place is empty, except for the hooded robes, blankets, and heaters looking for company. This is also when the bartenders serve steaming cocktails that take away the chill even faster than mom's chicken soup, which isn't usually served with a rooftop view. At night, little candles on the tables add even more magical sparkle to the Midtown skyline.

⌣ essentials

| 230 Fifth Avenue (at 27th Street), Manhattan 10001

(*C*) (212) 725-4300   (*✈*) 230-fifth.com

$ Free admission; cost varies according to drink and menu selection

(*☽*) Open daily, Monday–Friday, 4 p.m.–4 a.m.; Saturday–Sunday, 11 a.m.–4 a.m.

🚍 **By subway:** N, R, or W to 28th Street/Broadway; F, B, or D to 23rd Street/Sixth Avenue; 6 to 28th Street/Park Avenue.
By bus: M2 or 3 to Fifth Avenue/27th Street; M5, 6, or 7 to Broadway/27th Street.

peaceful place 121

UNNAMED ATRIUM
Midtown Manhattan

CATEGORY ︾ urban surprises ✪

*T*his is just a simple wide space between two skyscrapers that's been turned into an elongated plaza, with a curved transparent roof that acts as a radiator in winter, heat deflector in summer, and umbrella year-round. You could make believe that you are hiding between the cracks in the skyline, or, if you get a take-out espresso from a nearby coffee shop, that you are really sitting in Milan's Galleria. It's lined with bistro-type tables popular with office workers at lunchtime, so avoid the noon hour. In mid-morning and mid-afternoon, it's usually empty enough to find solitude, along with good light for reading. And great for sipping espresso.

︾ essentials

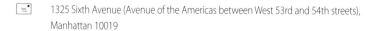

> 📧 1325 Sixth Avenue (Avenue of the Americas between West 53rd and 54th streets), Manhattan 10019

> 📞 No phone   🌐 No Web site $ Free admission

> 🕐 Monday–Sunday, 8 a.m.–7 p.m.

> 🚌 **By subway:** 1 to 50th Street; B, D, or E to Seventh Avenue.
> **By bus:** M50 to Sixth Avenue; M1, 2, 3, 4, 5, 6, or 7 to 53rd Street.

peaceful place 122

VAN CORTLANDT PARK
Riverdale and North Bronx, Bronx

CATEGORY ◡ parks & gardens ✪ ✪

oo bad the lovely lake dotted with ducks borders a municipal golf course with
golf cart activity and, behind that, the Major Deegan Expressway humming
with traffic noise. Avoid them all by heading over the little footbridge to the pond-size
north side of the lake, where a small waterfall masks the road noise. There's a gravel
path here, with a row of benches facing in alternating directions—this one toward the
lake, the next one toward the reeds and other marsh plants on the other side of the
path. The best access to the lake and wetlands area is between the wrought-iron fences
that ring the Revolutionary era Van Cortlandt House and the more modern Nature
Center, home to the park's Urban Rangers. A warning: This path starts out paved but
turns to uneven stones within 50 feet, so be sure to wear sturdy shoes. There are several
picnic tables here, too. The sturdy brick Van Cortlandt House Museum [Broadway at
West 246th Street, 10471, (718) 543-3344, vancortlandthouse.org] is well worth visiting for a peaceful interlude; it is the oldest house in the Bronx, with period furnishings
and family memorabilia.

◡ essentials

☷	Van Cortlandt Park South (West 240th Street) to Parkway North and the border with Westchester County, between Broadway and Jerome Avenue and Van Cortlandt Park East; Bronx 10471
✆	Friends of Van Cortlandt Park: (718) 601-1553; Urban Park Rangers: (718) 548-0912
✈	nycgovparks.org/parks/vancortlandtpark or vancortlandt.org

$ Free admission   🕐   Open daily, 6 a.m.–1 a.m.

🚍   **By subway:** 1 to 242nd Street (last stop); 4 to Woodlawn Avenue (last stop).
By bus: Bx9 along Broadway (western edge of park); Bx16, 31, or 34 (eastern edge of park).

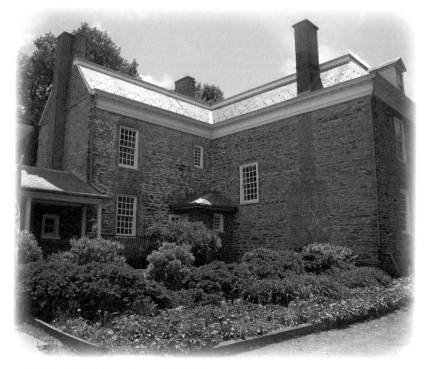

The Van Cortlandt House dates to Colonial times.

peaceful place 123

WASHINGTON SQUARE PARK
Lower Manhattan

CATEGORY ↙ parks & gardens ✪ ✪

he landmark marble 1892 Washington Arch, designed by architect Stanford White, marks the beginning of Fifth Avenue and is a photographer's favorite, along with the impeccable row of outrageously expensive Greek Revival houses on the park's northern border. This is a busy park at the heart of Greenwich Village—the backyard for students attending New York University and popular with local residents and street performers ranging from folk singers to acrobats. In nice weather it is almost impossible to find an empty bench or get a seat on the "lip" of the gigantic stone fountain that dominates the park's center. The only really quiet place is the area close to Waverly Place where chess players congregate—depending on the weather, a dozen or more regulars who hustle passersby for games—although the level of noise depends on the amount and volume of the kibitzing. But if you are wandering around the village, this is a must-visit. Just watch out for the skateboarders, bicyclists, Frisbee throwers, and running toddlers. Buy a couple of really good, high-quality hot dogs—generally voted as the best in NYC—and a papaya smoothie at Gray's Papaya [(212) 260-3532] on the corner of Sixth Avenue and Eighth Street, and turn your lap into a tailgate party.

↶ essentials

▣ West Fourth Street/Waverly Place between MacDougal Street and University Place, Manhattan 10003

☏ (212) 639-9675

🌐 nycgovparks.org/parks/washingtonsquarepark

$ Free admission

🕐 Open daily, sunrise to midnight

🚌 **By subway:** A, B, C, D, E, or F to West Fourth Street.

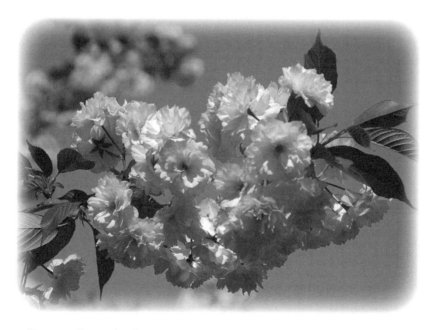

Cherry trees bloom each spring.

peaceful place 124

WAVE HILL
Riverdale, Bronx
CATEGORY ↝ scenic vistas ✪ ✪ ✪

*J*t's an "aha" moment when you walk through the tree-shaded entrance of this
garden and the vista pops open to reveal a huge, open lawn, the Hudson River,
and the black Palisades cliffs beyond it. Yes, the New York Botanical Garden in the Bronx
is more famous and ten times the size, which is exactly why this is my choice for solitude.
Grab one of the special simple wooden Wave Hill chairs sprinkled about, which you are
encouraged to move to suit your personal pleasure—sitting solo under a massive oak,

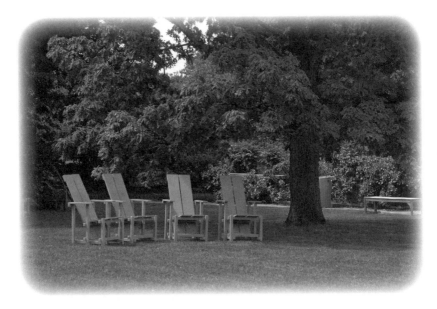

Wave Hill encourages visitors to linger.

one of the largest elms in New York City, or sunning yourself on one of the landscaped terraces, including the cafe terrace. This is the former estate of the fabulously wealthy Perkins family (George W. Perkins was a partner of J. P. Morgan), and prior to that, the Appleton family rented the house to such luminaries as Theodore Roosevelt's family when he was just a boy, as well as Mark Twain. One of the stately homes now features a lovely, sun-splashed art gallery with rotating exhibits on some theme of nature; when I visited recently, it was interpretations of the trees of Wave Hill. When to go? The flowers and foliage are different each season, and winter has a special appeal for the Technicolor early afternoon sunsets across the Hudson River. The English-style Wild Garden is lush from spring to fall, and the cacti-filled greenhouse is warm and toasty when it's cold outside. Wave Hill is least crowded on Friday mornings and most crowded on Tuesday and Saturday mornings, when it's free until noon.

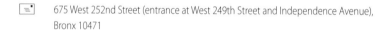

essentials

📧 675 West 252nd Street (entrance at West 249th Street and Independence Avenue), Bronx 10471

📞 (718) 549-3200   🌐 wavehill.org

$ Adults $8; seniors and students $4; children age 6 and up $2; free until noon on Tuesdays and Saturdays year-round and all day Tuesdays during January–April, July–August, and November–December

🕐 April 15–October 14: Tuesday–Sunday, and some holiday Mondays, 9 a.m.–5:30 p.m. October 15–April 14: Tuesday–Sunday, and some holiday Mondays, 9 a.m.–4:30 p.m.; June–July, to 8:30 p.m. on Wednesdays. (Greenhouses and galleries open at 10 a.m.)

🚌 **By subway:** 1 to West 242nd Street, then take the free shuttle service to and from Wave Hill; call or check the Web site for the shuttle schedule.
By bus: Take the BxM1 Express bus from Manhattan's East Side, or the BxM2 bus from Manhattan's West Side.
By train: Take the Metro-North train to Riverdale, then take the free shuttle service to and from Wave Hill; call or check the Web site for the shuttle schedule.

peaceful place 125

WESTERN PROMENADE, ROOSEVELT ISLAND
Roosevelt Island, Upper Manhattan

CATEGORY ✌ scenic vistas ✪ ✪ ✪

*A*lthough the promenade runs the length of the island, the section north of the tram is more accessible and close to one of my favorite spots, the Meditation Steps. The spectacular view across the East River to Manhattan is soul filling, especially when tugboats and pleasure boats polka dot the view. Then walk or take the island's red bus to the northern tip of this residential island community, on a spit of land between Queens and Manhattan, to Lighthouse Park, to admire an 1872 Gothic-style stone lighthouse built by the same architect who designed St. Patrick's Cathedral. And to admire the view, of course. You are less likely to find a secluded spot on warm-weather weekends, since this is the front yard for the island's residents.

✌ essentials

📧 Roosevelt Island Visitor Center, opposite tram dock, Roosevelt Island, Manhattan 10044

☎ (212) 688-4836   🌐 rioc.com $ Free admission

🕐 Visitor center: Saturday–Sunday, noon–5 p.m., winter;
Thursday–Sunday, noon–5 p.m., spring–fall

🚌 **By subway from Manhattan:** 4, 5, N, R, or W to Lexington Avenue/59th Street and walk east to take the tram at Second Avenue and 59th Street. **By bus:** Q32, M31, or M57 to Lexington Avenue/59th Street. **By subway from Queens:** F to Roosevelt Island; N,7, or W to Queensboro Plaza, then Q102 bus to Roosevelt Island.

peaceful place 126

WEST POND, JAMAICA BAY WILDLIFE REFUGE
Queens

CATEGORY ⌣ outdoor habitats ✪ ✪ ✪

ven though this is the more popular trail here, you are unlikely to pass more than a few fellow bird-watchers or hikers even on a warm-weather weekend. The most popular part of the trail is a wide gravel path with the open expanse of the marsh-ringed pond on one side and Jamaica Bay on the other. If you are lucky, you'll see the resident ospreys or their chicks flitting about the nest, which is close enough to the trail that you don't even need binoculars. My choice for repose, though, is to sit on one of the railroad-tie benches and watch the wine-red ibis and snow-white heron in the pond. There are picnic tables just behind the Nature Center at the entrance to the trail.

⌣ essentials

▣   Gateway National Recreation Area, Queens 11693

✆   (718) 318-4340

🌐   nps.gov/gate

$ Free admission

🕐   Visitor center: open daily, 8:30 a.m.–5 p.m. Trails open sunrise to sunset.

🚌   **By subway:** A train to Broad Channel Station; walk to Crossbay Boulevard and turn right (north) about a three-quarter mile to refuge.
By bus: Q21 or 53 to refuge.

peaceful place 127

WINTER GARDEN AND PLAZA, WORLD FINANCIAL CENTER

Lower Manhattan

CATEGORY ↲ scenic vistas ✪ ✪ ✪

*T*his soaring glass and marble atrium across the West Side Highway from the World Trade Center was shattered to pieces in the September 11, 2001, attack, and it was the first structure in the area to be rebuilt. It's a glorious, restful space, filled with benches, palm trees that are several stories tall, and light dancing through the greenhouselike space. In mid-morning and mid-afternoon, when office workers are not bustling through on their way to or from work or lunch, the semicircle of marble steps is my choice location here. I head there for its raised, almost bird's-eye view across the North Cove Harbor and the Hudson River. It's also the best spot for viewing the World Trade Center rebuilding—much better than trying to peer through the holes in the metal fence on the pedestrian overpass between the World Trade Center and the Winter Garden. My favorite spot, though, is the seemingly endless outdoor plaza alongside the Hudson River. The plaza is so big that even when it's crowded, it's not crowded.

↲ essentials

⌨ 220 Vesey Street, Manhattan 10281

☏ (212) 417-7000   ☝ worldfinancialcenter.com $ Free admission

🕓 Monday–Friday, 6 a.m.–10 p.m.; Saturday–Sunday, 7 a.m.–8 p.m.

By subway: A, C, J, M, Z, 1, 2, 3, 4, or 5 to Fulton Street/Broadway-Nassau;
E to World Trade Center.
By bus: M1 or 6 to Broadway and Liberty Street; M9 to South End Avenue;
M 20 or 22 to North End Avenue.

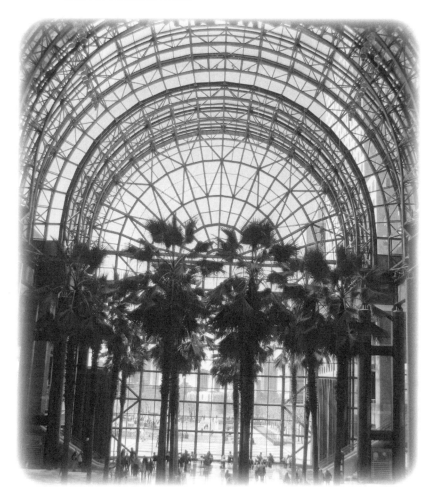

Palm trees punctuate the glass atrium.

peaceful place 128

YELO SPA
Midtown Manhattan

CATEGORY ⌣ shops & services ✪ ✪ ✪

*I*f you've ever wanted to take a power nap in the middle of the day, this is the place. Specially designed zero-gravity recliners in private spaces called cabins immerse you into the YeloNap. You'll experience gentle, changing colors and light, soothing sounds, and, unless you decline, aromatherapy. It feels something like a quick trip back to the womb. Except this place has 500-thread-count linens and soft cashmere blankets. You can combine your naptime experience with an add-on massage or facial. My vote is to have a treatment first and then become temporarily vegetative in totally relaxed bliss. Oh, sweet escape!

⌣ essentials

☰ 315 West 57th Street (between Eighth and Ninth avenues), Manhattan 10019

✆ (212) 245-8235   ✹ yelonyc.com $ Prices start at $15 for a 20-minute YeloNap

🕐 Open Monday–Friday, 10 a.m.–9 p.m.; Saturday, noon–8 p.m.; Sunday, noon–7 p.m.

🚌 **By subway:** 1, A, B, C, or D to 59th Street/Columbus Circle.
   By bus: M57 or 31 to Eighth Avenue; M10, 20, or 104 to 57th Street.

peaceful place 129

YESHIVA UNIVERSITY MUSEUM
Greenwich Village, Lower Manhattan
CATEGORY reading rooms ⚫ ⚫ ⚫

his is the smallest of New York City's three Jewish museums, and because it is part of a university, there is a strong educational component. Not even the section where scholars pore over ancient prayer books and manuscripts is what I would call a fancy library, but it is definitely hushed. The windows of the bookshop overlook a pretty tree-lined block. The galleries focus on the art and culture of 3,000 years of Jewish history, ranging from ceremonial and household objects to contemporary art by Jewish artists from around the world. There is also a small but charming sculpture garden and a wonderful children's book area.

essentials

15 West 16th Street (between Fifth and Sixth avenues inside Center for Jewish History), Manhattan 10011

(212) 294-8330   yumuseum.org

$ Adults $8; seniors and students $6; free for members and children under age 5; free Monday, Wednesday (5 p.m.–8 p.m.), and Friday

Sunday, Tuesday, and Thursday, 11 a.m.–5 p.m.; Monday, 3:30 p.m.–8 p.m.; Wednesday, 11 a.m.–8 p.m.; Friday, 11 a.m.–2:30 p.m.

By subway: A, B, C, D, E, F, 1, 2, or 3 to 14th Street; L, N, Q, R, W, 4, 5, or 6 to Union Square. **By bus:** M2, 3, 5, 6, or 7 to Fifth/Madison Avenue to 14th Street.

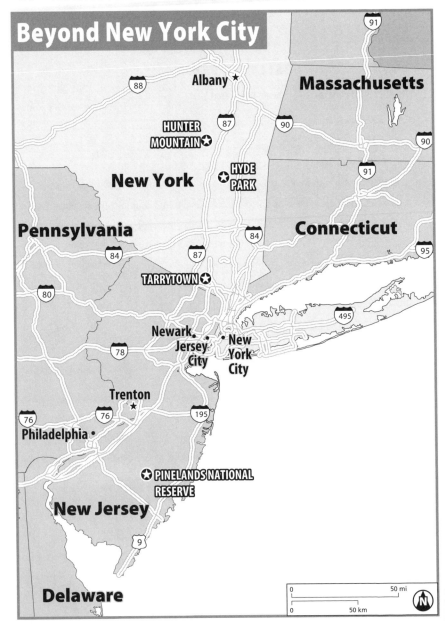

Beyond New York City

Massachusetts

Albany

HUNTER MOUNTAIN

New York

HYDE PARK

Pennsylvania

Connecticut

TARRYTOWN

Newark
Jersey City

New York City

Trenton

Philadelphia

PINELANDS NATIONAL RESERVE

New Jersey

Delaware

0   50 mi
0   50 km

bonus section: beyond new york city

*I*n my opinion, shared by many, New York City has more of everything than any other place in the world. That includes more peaceful surprises. But sometimes you just have to leave town for a change of scenery, even if it's only for a day. Here are my choices for a brief escape, all within two to three hours' driving time from Times Square—depending on traffic, or the train or bus schedule. You can enjoy any one of these four destinations in a day, or turn the jaunt into a leisurely weekend retreat. If you decide to stay overnight, you'll find many family-owned bed-and-breakfasts close by. You may note that I have rated all four of these sites as three stars for peacefulness.

HUNTER MOUNTAIN
Hunter, New York
CATEGORY ↵ outdoor habitats ✪ ✪ ✪

*M*y idea of serenity in winter is speeding downhill on my skis, shutting out the world and its problems by concentrating on every snowflake and turn. I learned to ski here, and so did my kids. Even before that, my parents and I vacationed near here each summer when this was a lively part of the legendary Catskills Borscht Belt. Hunter Mountain simply has the best snow and the best terrain, from gentle groomers to challenging steeps, within 150 miles of Midtown Manhattan. The chairlifts run in summer and fall as well, when hikers and mountain bikers own the trails. There's also a state park nearby, in Haines Falls, with yet more hiking trails, and a lake for canoeing and fishing. Other than winter, my favorite time here is autumn, when the air is as crisp as a local apple, and the mountain is dressed in a wardrobe of reds and gold. In winter, several sports shops run day-trip ski bus shuttles to the slopes from Penn Station, and it's common to see people like me carrying their skis on the subway to meet the bus. In other seasons, you can take the Adirondack Trailways bus between the Port Authority Terminal and Hunter. (800) 486-8376, huntermtn.com

HYDE PARK, NEW YORK

CATEGORY ⌣ historic sites, outdoor habitats, parks & gardens, scenic vistas, enchanting walks ✪ ✪ ✪

*A*s you can see from the category selections above, this destination has it all! The Roosevelt family had ties to the Hudson River Valley dating back to the 17th century, settling in Hyde Park in the 1800s. Hyde Park is the site of the Franklin D. Roosevelt Home, Library and Museum. Franklin and Eleanor Roosevelt are buried in the rose garden between the greenhouse and the library, from which he sometimes delivered his legendary wartime fireside chats. After the death of the Roosevelts' neighbor, Frederick Vanderbilt, that estate was also donated to the National Park Service and is now the Vanderbilt Mansion National Historic Site. I am always blown away by Louise Vanderbilt's bedroom, modeled and decorated like that of Marie Antoinette's room in Versailles, although all that fussy gold detail does not seem restful to my eyes.

A few miles south is the campus of the Culinary Institute of America, the "other" CIA, which has trained many of the top chefs in the United States. There are several first-class restaurants on campus, all student-staffed, including the formal French Escoffier, but I prefer to get a take-out picnic lunch from the cafe and sit on one of the grassy lawns overlooking the Hudson River and Valley, especially at sunset.

Franklin D. Roosevelt National Historic Site: (800) 337-8474, nps.gov/hofr

Vanderbilt Mansion National Historic Site: (845) 229-9115, nps.gov/vama

Culinary Institute of America: (845) 452-9600, ciachef.edu

KYKUIT AND SUNNYSIDE
Tarrytown, New York

CATEGORY ↵ historic sites, enchanting walks ✪ ✪ ✪

*T*he Tarrytown area has attracted homeowners—from the original Dutch settlers in the 1600s to the Rockefellers in the 1800s to today's commuters—for its Hudson River views and proximity to Manhattan. Kykuit (pronounced KYE-cut and the Dutch word for "look-out") is a stately, vine-covered Beaux Arts mansion. It housed four generations of Rockefellers, including Nelson, the four-term New York governor and U.S. vice president. The mansion and its gardens are filled with museum-quality art, including works by Pablo Picasso, Henry Moore, and Alexander Calder. Nelson's mother, Abby Aldrich Rockefeller, wife of John D. Jr., was one of the founders of NYC's Museum of Modern Art. Guided tours of the mansion and garden, where you can enjoy the hilltop views of the Hudson River and valley, are offered.

Also visit Philipsburg Manor, just down the hill, which is now a living-history farm, with vegetables and historical breeds of livestock reflecting life in the 18th century.

You'll need an additional day to add on nearby Sunnyside—home of Washington Irving, who wrote "Rip Van Winkle" and "The Legend of Sleepy Hollow" about this area—and the Sleepy Hollow Cemetery, where you'll find Irving's grave. You can also see grave sites of Andrew Carnegie, Walter Chrysler, and Brooke and Vincent Astor. Best of all, you can get here on a relaxed ride on the Metro-North commuter train. (914) 631-8200 (Monday–Friday); (914) 631-3992 (Saturday–Sunday); historichudsonvalley.com.

NEW JERSEY PINELANDS NATIONAL RESERVE

Pine Barrens, New Jersey

CATEGORY ↵ outdoor habitats, enchanting walks ✪ ✪ ✪

*F*rom blueberry picking in summer to scary Halloween moonlight hikes, to canoeing, kayaking, and hiking in between, the Pine Barrens is a multi-faceted place—covering seven counties and more than 1.1 million acres of land—approximately 100 miles south of Manhattan and 30 miles east of Philadelphia. For scenic paddling, try the Mullica River, where you can enjoy in solitude the dense holly, pines, and oaks, and the mallards and egrets you'll see in great numbers. Since I'm not a fisherwoman, I can't tell you the best spots for largemouth bass. A perfect second day for me is wandering the dunes, kicking the sand on the Jersey seashore, and watching the occasional surfer dude glide over the waves. If you plan on staying overnight, there are more than a dozen towns located reasonably nearby. (609) 894-7300; nps.gov/pine or pineypower.com

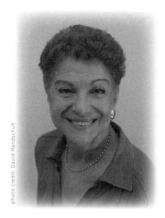

photo credit: David Handschuh

*A*uthor and photographer Evelyn Kanter is a citizen of the world: You can find her scuba diving with sharks in the Caribbean, white-water rafting in South America, hiking among ancient temples in the Far East, or speeding down a ski slope somewhere. That is Kanter's lifestyle, and what she has written about for publications including *The New York Times, Travel & Leisure*, and airline in-flight magazines. But such meanderings always lead this native and lifelong New York City resident back to her own Manhattan neighborhood. She welcomed the opportunity to launch Peaceful Places with her hometown as the first title in this new metropolitan series.* It is her latest book after *Eating the Hudson Valley: A Food Lover's Guide to Local Wineries, Dining, & More*, widely regarded as the definitive resource on the region that is New York City's northern neighbor. With the heart and soul of New York in her genes—plus a career as a newspaper and broadcast news reporter, magazine writer, book author, and Web site blogger—Kanter serves up a unique collection of remarkable and tranquil urban escapes in *Peaceful Places: New York City*.

Peaceful Places: Los Angeles, by Laura Randall, premieres in mid-2010.